NURSING PROFILE

NURSING PROFILE

Cecy Correia
Nursing Tutor
Uday General School of Nursing
Cardinal Gracias Memorial Hospital
Sandor, Bangli, Vasai (W)
Thane (Maharashtra), India

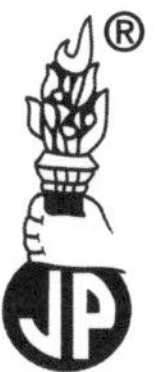

JAYPEE BROTHERS MEDICAL PUBLISHERS (P) LTD

Mumbai • St Louis (USA) • Panama City (Panama) • London (UK)
New Delhi • Ahmedabad • Bengaluru • Chennai • Hyderabad • Kochi
Kolkata • Lucknow • Nagpur

Published by
Jitendar P Vij
Jaypee Brothers Medical Publishers (P) Ltd

Corporate Office
4838/24 Ansari Road, Daryaganj, **New Delhi** - 110002, India
Phone: +91-11-43574357, Fax: +91-11-43574314

Registered Office
B-3 EMCA House, 23/23B Ansari Road, Daryaganj, **New Delhi** - 110 002, India
Phones: +91-11-23272143, +91-11-23272703, +91-11-23282021, +91-11-23245672
Rel: +91-11-32558559, Fax: +91-11-23276490, +91-11-23245683
e-mail: jaypee@jaypeebrothers.com, Website: www.jaypeebrothers.com

Offices in India

- **Ahmedabad**, Phone: Rel: +91-79-32988717, e-mail: ahmedabad@jaypeebrothers.com
- **Bengaluru**, Phone: Rel: +91-80-32714073, e-mail: bangalore@jaypeebrothers.com
- **Chennai**, Phone: Rel: +91-44-32972089, e-mail: chennai@jaypeebrothers.com
- **Hyderabad**, Phone: Rel:+91-40-32940929, e-mail: hyderabad@jaypeebrothers.com
- **Kochi**, Phone: +91-484-2395740, e-mail: kochi@jaypeebrothers.com
- **Kolkata**, Phone: +91-33-22276415, e-mail: kolkata@jaypeebrothers.com
- **Lucknow**, Phone: +91-522-3040554, e-mail: lucknow@jaypeebrothers.com
- **Mumbai**, Phone: Rel: +91-22-32926896, e-mail: mumbai@jaypeebrothers.com
- **Nagpur**, Phone: Rel: +91-712-3245220, e-mail: nagpur@jaypeebrothers.com

Overseas Offices

- **North America Office, USA,** Ph: 001-636-6279734
  e-mail: jaypee@jaypeebrothers.com, anjulav@jaypeebrothers.com
- **Central America Office, Panama City, Panama**
  Ph: 001-507-317-0160, e-mail: cservice@jphmedical.com
  Website: www.jphmedical.com
- **Europe Office, UK,** Ph: +44 (0) 2031708910
  e-mail: info@jpmedpub.com

Nursing Profile

© 2011, Jaypee Brothers Medical Publishers

This book has been published in good faith that the material provided by author is original. Every effort is made to ensure accuracy of material, but the publisher, printer and author will not be held responsible for any inadvertent error(s). In case of any dispute, all legal matters are to be settled under Delhi jurisdiction only.

First Edition: **2011**
ISBN 978-93-5025-159-1
Typeset at JPBMP typesetting unit
Printed at Rajkamal Electric Press, Plot No. 2, Phase-IV, Kundli, Haryana.

To

Anthony Gonzalves
who was a born teacher and has spent his life
in teaching career
and believed
that education is the only thing that will
change the face of the society.
May who read this book
be inspired and blessed.

Preface

The book as it is titled *Nursing Profile* and med-surge is a practical and comprehensive. During my teaching and evaluation, I felt the need for these topics that are not only important to student who have to submit there assignments but also equally important for nursing teachers to revise and use as an aid to guide the students in their theory and practical.

Therefore, this book is not only important to nursing students but also nursing tutors as well. It is prepared in simple manner for all to understand and use. In addition, students are always very anxious to understand and complete the cases. Therefore, I thought of putting them in the form of a book which will be useful for their reference. It will enhance nurses in field area and in clinical area for direction.

There are some pictures to give an idea for the students to prepare a variety of project exhibition; on different topics, they can select after understanding the main idea. These were the topics I had prepared with my students and experience, the effectiveness and usefulness for the public health, motivation and awareness; and the results were very positive.

This book has its own style and importance. I am sure the teachers and the students will find it very useful in their studies and guidance for better function in carrying out their responsibilities.

Modern health care delivery system has become complex and there is a need for updated information. It will help to improve the skills or levels of knowledge so that she can be better equipped. Taking the responsibilities for oneself is the key to successful health promotion. The possibilities are endless and the opportunities are countless. In fact, for a nurse with drive and ambition, the world is truly not enough.

Knowledgeable nursing services are indispensable. Applying and teaching all we know for patient's highest potential for healthful living. As she is the key person and the backbone of the health care delivery system, she is a pillar on which modern care is based, where she has diverse roles and responsibilities to fulfill.

What will be the pattern of future health work?
With profound changes that impose heavier burdens on , continuous professional development, to exploit advances, greater work specialization and high skill growing demand by consumer preferences and new technologies, nursing is key drive. How can new and effective educational methods be introduced and strengthened in nursing practice, as the nurse's role is in the spotlight more than ever before.

Today, curriculum is reviewed, revised and restructured for improving the quality of human life. As a hungry man needs food and water, so the sick man needs nursing care and the nurse is a mediator.

The word guru means dispeller of darkness. Guru removes ignorance and gives light of knowledge and wisdom. The combinations of teacher's wisdom and the energy of the students to go forward making a vibrant progressive body of healthy society.

May this book bring blessings to all who read and use it for service of humankind.

Cecy Correia

———— Acknowledgments ————

'Destiny is not a matter of chance, it is a matter of choice'. The greatest thing in life is to keep your mind alert and attune to new knowledge and information. Toil for it. Train your mind towards it. Tap your individual capacities. Be prepared to face your professional skill with advanced globalization fast paced in competitive world, where you require excellent academic record to overcome adverse circumstances. We are what we repeatedly do. Be the master of your own destiny.

I express my thanks to my husband, Alois, for his continuous support and encouragement.

I extend my gratitude to nursing school and my students who motivated me to write this book.

I am grateful to Jaypee Brothers Medical Publishers for their high standard, and quick working strategies. They have exceptional quality services, I was impressed. They are excellent and I am privileged having them as my publisher. They have boosted my self-confidence and will power. It is because of their constant encouragement, I was able to proceed with this work. It is my great pleasure to know them. They are unique and they stand out distinctly. They deserve my heart-felt thanks from the bottom of my heart for helping me to realize my dream of writing the book. Gratitude is attitude of life which flows from my heart to the publishing house.

Through their medical publishing, they have tried to give the best of quality books over the years. It will help coping up in profound changes occurring in nursing and in health care delivery to give skillful continuous knowledge for today's nurses.

Contents

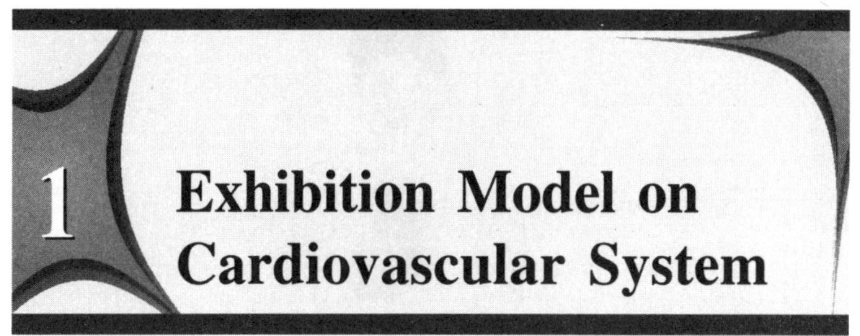

FORM OF PROJECT: MODEL OF HEART EXHIBITION

In 21st century, media is playing major role, technology has made possible such sweeping advances in communication. A popular saying, "I hear, I forge, I see, I remember, I do, I understand."

Model enhances clarity in communication and enriches learning. It provides direct, concrete, and purposeful experience; it gives opportunity to touch, to feel, to see a model. It brings remote events of either space or time in classroom. Suitable topic covered by such learning helps to increase retention and motivation, it stimulates discussion.

Model is a life-size miniature substitute for real things which is concrete object made up of clay, pulp, plaster of Paris, cotton, cardboard, thermocole, cloth, wood, etc.

EXPLANATION OF CORONARY ANGIOPLASTY

Health education through its process which effects changes in the health practices of the people. It is a knowledge and information related to bringing change in the attitudes. To have a good health is an invaluable asset, which helps people to solve their problems by their own way. To create awareness and motivate change, this type of health education is like cement, which binds together the bricks which makes people

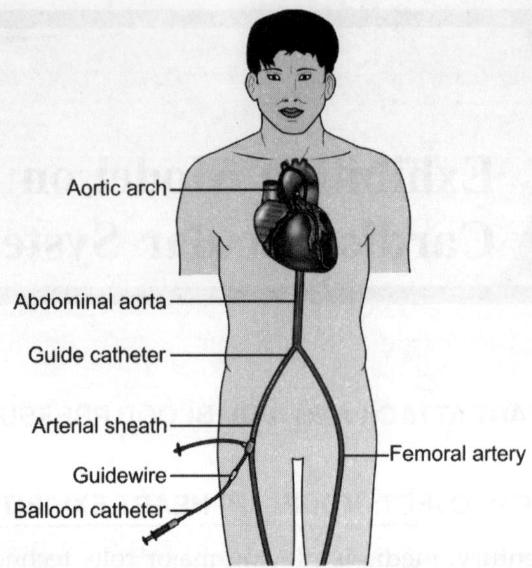

Fig. 1.1: Coronary angioplasty

to think for themselves. Ignorance can be removed by such education (Fig. 1.1).

It helps in meaningful learning. It concretizes abstract concepts. It enlarges objects to an observable size. It provides correct concept of a real object. It promotes creative interest among pupil.

Cross-sectional model, e.g. of blood vessel, working model, e.g. fetal circulation too can be made in a similar way.

Types of Project

Portable and can be assembled after dismantling and shifted easily.
1. Name of the Institution
2. Year of student
3. Name of the member
   a.
   b.
   c.

   d.

   e.

   f.

   g.

4. Date of commencement
5. Date of completion of project
6. Name of teacher

Need for the Project

- As people living in the rural areas have no idea about the diseases related to heart, therefore, they neglect the signs and symptoms occurring in their body.
- To prevent all the complications, which becomes a risk factor for the people?
- Which can be fatal to their life?
- How smoking and alcohol affect heart diseases?
- How diet affects?
- How physical inactivity affects?
- How stress and anxiety affect?
- To prevent all these, we have come together as a group and get all the needed information about diseases of cardiovascular diseases.
- Especially heart attack and high blood pressure. So that they can be provided with enough knowledge and can live their life happily and safely with our effort, tips, and education.

Planning of the Project

- Models
- Interiors of the heart
- Systemic circulation of the blood
- Signs and symptoms
- Risk factors
- Prevention
- Diet
- Charts of hypertension and stress
- Slogans

- Skit
- Exercise for a healthier heart
- Jagruti songs.

Specimens were taken from real objects taken from the natural setting, which makes instruction more meaningful, vivid and impressive. Model arouses interest, involves all five senses, develops observation skills and makes teaching lively.

UNDERSTANDING OF ANATOMY, PHYSIOLOGY AND THE FUNCTIONS OF HEART

Group Reflection

- What is the purpose of the project?
- What are you/people suppose to learn?
- What skills are you suppose to capture?
- How will you decide project work in the field?
- What are you suppose to produce?

Preplan

The incidence of coronary heart disease (CHD) is increasing with a galloping speed and unless active, preventive and curative measures are taken it will soon assume epidemic proportions.

In the last two decades, there have been revolutionary advances in the management of heart diseases. Nevertheless, it is important to be familiar with symptoms, preventive measures and methodology of management of these devastating diseases. With this in mind, we, as a group, presented this project. So that the people have insight in this very important area of public health.

We decided to explain the structure of the heart (Fig. 1.2). We made a heart model, then we divided it into pieces for different groups. We plan to explain first the definition, causes, signs and symptoms, prevention, diet and treatment. We plan to perform a skit through which the simple people can understand the risk factors and early detection of heart diseases. We plan to make slogans for better understanding

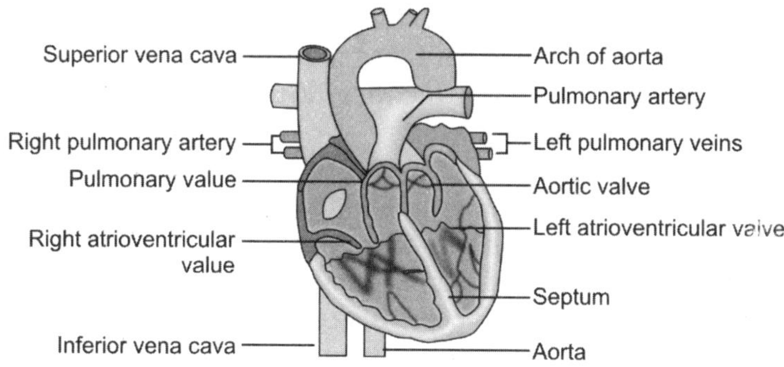

Fig. 1.2: Structure of heart

and remembrance of certain obvious signs and risk factors that are common in emergency to save life.

We plan to take blood pressure of few people and showed them in demonstration.

We also demonstrated artificial respiration, heart massage, by demonstrating first aid measures.

Background Information of the Area through Detailed Survey

Gathered all the Information by Meeting and Interviewing the Family Members

Past history of the disease conditions and the heavy smokers special interview, etc. we got to know that members of many different families had been affected with different cardiac diseases mainly hypertension and massive heart arrest. Due to lack of knowledge related to hypertension and cardiac arrest, we as a teamly, came forward to take up this challenge and prepare the exhibition and educating people with adequate information regarding the same.

Goals and Objectives

1. To reach out to the people and give knowledge about heart disease in a simplest and easier way

2. To give systematic step-by-step information through different charts and parts of model
3. To give two different pictures of persons with healthy heart and unhealthy heart
4. To give information on preventing factors
5. To prevent information of early diagnosis and treatment
6. To give information of appropriate diet and exercise
7. To find out any hereditary family history
8. To detect congenital heart diseases
9. To find other diseases like thematic fever, etc. leading to heart disease
10. To explain the heart anatomy, its functions and vital importance
11. Do's and don'ts
12. Changing in your lifestyles
13. Follow-up care and regular medication
14. Tips for healthy heart
15. Rest and relaxation
16. Investigations and diagnosis.

Collection of Data

Textbooks of medical, magazine articles, internet, information from survey done, PHC cases recorded, etc.

Assessment of Resources

We had tapped the low cost and locally available sufficient resources in order to start our project by explaining different systematic question supported by appropriate charts and models.

Fixing the Priority

We fixed the priority on the bases of survey and background information we had collected.

We also fixed as our priority to explain heart attack and high blood pressure among other cardiovascular diseases as it affected people and needed vital knowledge.

To increase public awareness and promoting the preventing measures to reduce such diseases, we fixed the priority.

Expected Outcome of the Project

We expected that people get motivated and become aware of their own health and health risks.

- That people develop healthy lifestyle and healthy habits.
- That people eat wholesome food and do activity and exercises.
- That people give up vices of smoking cigarettes, tobacco and alcohol.
- That people reduce the stress of life by accepting this in a positive way.
- That people understand the signs and symptoms of heart attack and rush the patient to the causality without wasting time.
- That people control there blood pressure by healthy living and get regular treatment.
- That people live healthy and happy life with health awareness.

HEART DISEASES ARE PUBLIC HEALTH PROBLEMS: TOGETHER HOW TO SOLVE THE PROBLEM— BY MOTIVATION AND AWARENESS IN THE PUBLIC

That people understand what we wanted to communicate with charts, posters, skits, jagruti songs, models and slogans (Fig. 1.3).

Implementation

Implementation done as the resources available and the target group that was present. Implemented as a team had preplanned keeping the time and place and priority in for front.

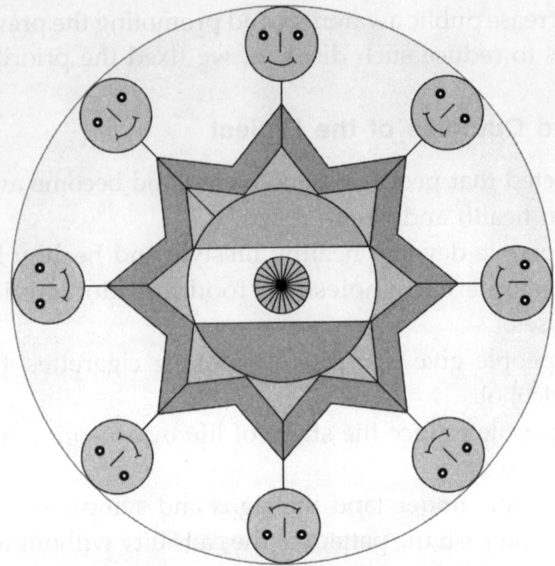

Fig. 1.3: Working together for health

Manpowered Required

Group of seven working united with local volunteers.

Equipment Required

Simple equipment that we had collected and preplanned with BP apparatus and stethoscope too was used.

Appropriate Technology

Verbally explanation, demonstration, skits, songs, models, charts, etc.

Organization—through help and cooperation of PHC and local people's help in rural field.

Schedule of Stages—Start to Finish

- 5.00 pm reached to the spot and displayed all the charts and necessary preparation

- 5.30 pm went to visit the nearby people for reminding them of the same
- 6.00 pm started our exhibition with an interaction and welcoming people and making them comfortable and preparing conducive atmosphere
- 6.30 pm controlling and as allotted the responsibility to the team started explanation of heart structure, blood circulation, signs and symptoms, diet, prevention, disease conditions, etc.
- 7.30 pm we concluded with feedback and people's reaction to it.

Educational Values of the Project

It was satisfying that we made some start towards public health problem of cardiovascular diseases and its prevention. It would remain as lasting impression with a difference of health education which was creative and not boring with variation.

We explained how blood circulates through the heart. Blood returns from all parts of the body to right side of the heart; from there, it is pumped to the lungs, where it drops carbon dioxide and picks up oxygen.

Group Presentation

Introduction

The concept of World Health Day was initiated by the World Heart Federation in conjunction with 'WHO', 'UNESCO' and United Nations with the purpose of increasing public awareness and promoting preventive measures to reduce cardiovascular diseases, e.g. high blood pressure, heart attack, stroke.

Heart diseases are world's largest killers, claiming 17.5 million lives per year. With hectic and changing lifestyle, heart disease has become the number one health priority of a nation.

Increasingly, we are seeing more and more patients, especially younger age group with coronary heart disease. This has an alarming fact.

An estimated 50 million Indians suffer from coronary artery disease. We claim to be vegetarians, but consume unimaginable amounts of fat as ghee and oils. Sedentary lifestyles, lack of exercise, smoking and use of tobacco in alternative forms like 'gutka', snuff and chewed tobacco abound in our society.

This exhibition will guide on how to look after your heart while it is functioning normally or even if you have heart disease by adopting a healthier lifestyle.

Know your heart and work towards making healthier. Believe that only a healthy heart will make healthy nation.

This project will help people understand their heart, and how to cope with its problems.

The human heart is a marvelous organ. Its function is to move the living stream of blood through all parts of the body, never stopping even for a moment in its endless activity. Your heart does an enormous amount of work. It beats over one hundred thousand times a day, continually pumping the blood through more than 60,000 miles of tiny blood vessels. These tiny capillaries are only a tenth of an inch long, but if they could be placed end-to-end, they would reach two and a half times around the earth at the equator. To maintain the right pressure, all these vessels must be filled with the right amount of blood; otherwise, the tissues of the body would waste away and die.

Short explanation and flash cards on each prepared:
- How the heart beats
- How the heart grows
- Circulation before birth
- Congenital heart diseases
- The blood circulation system
- Rheumatic heart disease
- Tools to examine the heart
- Heart check periodically.

Anatomy and Physiology of the Heart

The heart is a strong fist-sized muscle situated in the center of your chest and tilted a little to the left. It pumps blood through the blood vessels thereby delivering oxygen and nutrients to all parts of the body. The heart has four chambers, the ventricles, are the pumping chambers, which tirelessly perform the actual work of pumping blood: 60 to 90 times a minute, 24 hours a day, for as long as you live. During an average lifetime, the average heart beats over two billion times.

A thick band of muscle, the septum, separates the heart into two sets of pumps, the left and the right. Each side has a different function in the heart's pumping action. Like all tissues in the body, the heart requires oxygen-filled blood in order to function. Blood goes to nourish the heart through the tubes called coronary arteries.

The heart muscle needs oxygen-rich blood to function and oxygen-depleted blood must be carried away.

Coronary Arteries

Lifelines of the heart—although the heart is bathed in blood, it cannot derive its own nutrition from the blood it is continuously pumping. Atherosclerosis is the process of hardening of the coronary arteries.

INFORMATION DOCTORS CAN GET WITH ECG OF YOUR HEART

The Information that Doctor Gets from ECG Results

1. If any part of your heart is receiving less blood
2. If part of your heart muscle is damaged
3. If the muscles of your heart is thickened as can occur if you have high blood pressure
4. If any part of your heart is enlarged
5. If the valves of your heart are normal
6. Whether you have: hole; in your heart

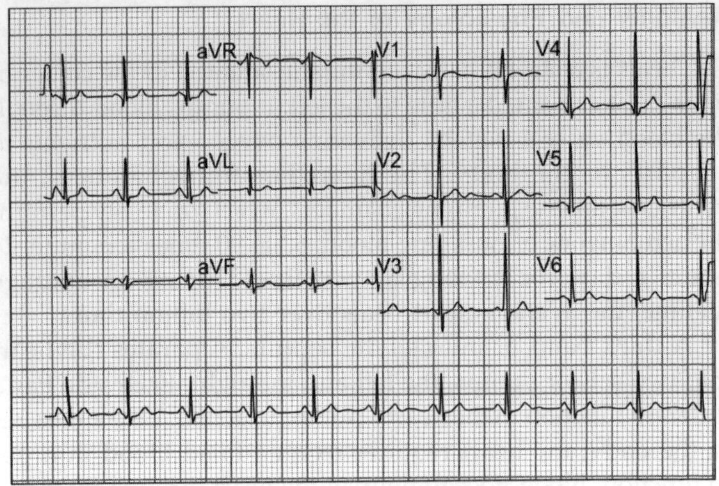

Fig. 1.4: Electrocardiogram

7. If the rhythm of your heart is normal, or irregular
8. The effect of certain medications on your heart
9. Whether the composition of salts in your body is normal
10. If it is inflamed, or if there is fluid within the pericardium.

Risk Factors for Heart Diseases

Major Risk Factors

Hypertension—high blood pressure increases your risk of heart disease, heart attack, and stroke. If you are obese, you smoke, have high cholesterol, your risk increases:
- High blood cholesterol
- Diabetes
- Obesity and overweight
- Smoking
- Physical inactivity
- Your gender
- Heredity
- Age.

Contributing risk factors:
- Stress
- Sex hormones
- Birth control pills
- Alcohol.

What is a Heart Attack?

The consequence of atherosclerosis, cholesterol somewhat like scales forming on the inside to a pipe with that inside artery gets narrowed, impeding normal blood flow, which comes with pain, which is dangerous, if blood clot formed at this, narrowed segment, it results in a shutting off the blood supply to part of the heart muscle. This part of the heart muscle gets damaged, resulting in a heart attack.

1. Intense discomfort in the chest, arm, back or jaw
2. The discomfort worsens with exertion
3. This pain lasts longer than the discomfort of angina, and is not relieved by rest or nitroglycerine
4. The pain may be associated with a sense of impending doom, severe weakness, dizziness, sweating, nausea, vomiting, breathlessness, fainting or palpitation.

Common Mistakes Committed During a Heart Attack

1. If I wait, may be the pain will go away. This is a very common mistake and results in the waste of valuable time. In the case of the heart, every minute counts. Time saved means heart muscles saved.
2. It is only gas—or acidity and attempts at self-medication with cold milk or antacids, further wasting time.
3. I will wait till morning—this can prove to be a serious mistake.
4. I cannot be having a heart attack—some people do not think they are the types who can have a heart attack and deny the possibility of a heart attack.

What to do During a Suspected Heart Attack?

1. Stop whatever you are doing.
2. Lie down and take a tablet of nitroglycerine. If the pain does not go away, you may take up to three tablets. If the pain still persists, you can be certain you are having a heart attack.
3. Tell someone what is happening, even if it is the middle of the night.
4. Take a tablet of soluble aspirin dissolved in water.
5. Call a doctor who will assess your condition and take an ECG.
6. If a doctor is not immediately available to take ECG, it is a good idea to go to the casualty of the nearest hospital or nursing home.
7. Remember time is crucial, minutes saved equals muscle saved.

How to Reduce Blood Cholesterol?

Lowering your blood cholesterol will reduce the rate of build-up of fatty substances in your coronary artery. This in turn will reduce your risk of a heart attack and death. There are three ways to lower blood cholesterol. Diet, exercise and weight loss and drug.

Take Diet that is low in saturated fats and cholesterol.

This diet has to continue for life and you will discover that such a diet will soon become your regular routine.

Reduce food intake and eat more fiber like fruits, vegetables, whole grain, beans, etc. A high fiber diet reduces the absorption of fats and cholesterol from the intestine. Reduce coffee or tea, and alcohol in moderation. Reduce fat intake, choose oils containing unsaturated fats in cooking. Use nonstick cookware, which reduces the requirement of oil in cooking. Never deep fry your food. When eating out, choose dishes that are broiled, baked, steamed or grilled rather than fried.

- Intake of garlic 30 gm per day is preferable.
- Intake of 2-3 teaspoon of oil per day is recommended.
- Foods are not good or bad.
- Tell me what you eat and I will tell you what you are.
- Quit smoking—tobacco smoke contains over 4,000 poisons and chemicals.
- Prevention is always better than cure.
- Smoking is suicide in slow motion.
- A cigarette is a white stick with a fire at one end and a fool at the other.
- The only way to stop smoking is—just stop—no ifs, ands or buts.
- Stress is the modern epidemic.

FOODS TO AVOID

Diet to be Avoided—Diet to be Taken in High Cholesterol, High Blood Pressure

- Organ meats, kidney, brain, liver
- Beef, veal, pork
- Oyster, clams, lobster, shrimp
- Sausages, salami, corned beef, chicken skin
- Whole milk, condensed milk, Bengali sweets
- Cream, butter, lard, cheese
- Khoya
- Egg yolk
- Mayonnaise, salad dressing
- Hydrogenated oils, ghee, coconut oil, palm oil
- Cream-filled biscuits, croissants
- Nuts
- Pastries, puddings
- Ice cream
- French fries

Foods to Eat

- Fruits, vegetables, salads
- Cereals, pulses

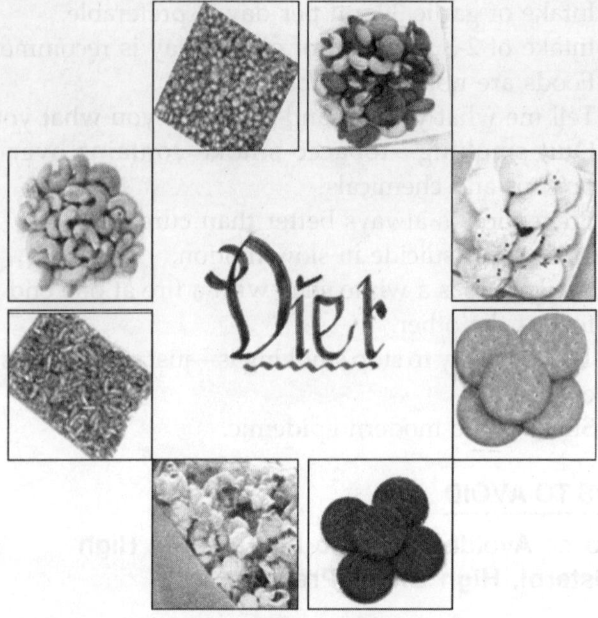

Fig. 1.5: Diet to eat

- Egg white
- Skim milk
- Cottage cheese
- Curd
- Chutneys, pickles with no oil
- Tea, coffee, fruit juice
- Potatoes, rice
- Almonds, walnuts
- Occasionally chicken without skin or fish not fried.

Even if you are already been diagnosed with heart disease, making lifestyle changes can help you live a longer, healthier and more enjoyable life, small easily achievable adaptations such as becoming more active in your everyday life and learning to enjoy fresh, wholesome food can make a tremendous difference to your well-being and improve the health of your heart.

Exercises—It is a physical activity in a form of exercise. Visit your physician before you start any exercise program. What sort of exercise is good for you? How much exercise, how long, how often? How much should I walk? Take precaution before starting.

For all-round fitness, do aerobic, resistance training and flexibility, e.g. walking, running, swimming, etc. and maintaining ideal weight are equally important for reducing high blood cholesterol. Becoming more active helps to reduce your blood pressure, improves your cholesterol level and by boosting your metabolism, helps control your weight, which reduces heart risk.

When you start exercising, your body' systems start working harmoniously together. Exercise enhances the body's ability to utilize oxygen more efficiently. Lungs expand, blood vessels open up, prevents formation of blood clot, body well-tuned engine works better and energy is expected to last longer.

Make exercise a way of life.

Without exercise, your body and mind suffers. You feel tired, restless and tense.

BENEFITS OF EXERCISE

Maintaining Weight and the Dangers of Over Weight on Health

1. Weight control
2. Lowered cholesterol
3. Reduced blood pressure
4. Less risk of having a heart attack
5. Faster recovery from heart attack
6. Control of blood sugar
7. Strong bones
8. Relaxation
9. Positive approach towards life, lesser stress
10. Better sleep

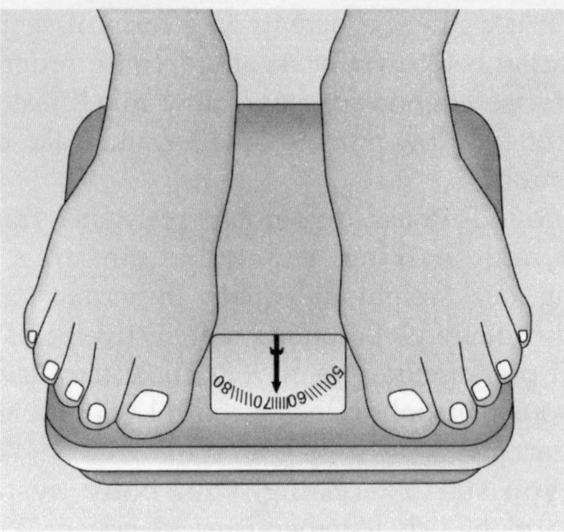

Fig. 1.6: Measuring the weight

11. Improved posture
12. Feeling fitter and stronger
13. Better digestion
14. Increased lifespan.

If you experience any of the following during exercising, consult your doctor. Chest pain, dizziness, light-headedness or confusion, nausea or vomiting, cramps-like pains in the legs, pale or bluish skin, breathlessness lasting for more than 10 minutes, palpitation, rapid or irregular heart beat, fluid retention that is swollen ankles, sudden weight gain.

Excuses not to do exercise—I have no time, I am too old, I am on my feet all day, I am exercising enough, I find exercising too boring, I am not the sporting type, I find exercise too strenuous, I cannot keep it up, it is too expensive, it could be dangerous.

Are You a Little Unfit?

- Do you get a little breathless on climbing those extra floors or carrying that extra weight?
- Has your energy diminished with age?

- Does your belly protrude a little too much, or do your muscles feel too flabby?
- Take the stairs instead of the lift, walk an extra bus stop before and after work, do not drive when you can walk.
- Choose an exercise that you like. It is easier to keep up.
- Gradually increase the intensity and frequency over weeks to months.
- A 5-minute cooling down period after exercising.
- Try it at the same everyday.
- Do not over do it.
- Avoid extreme heat or cold.
- Not after meals or alcohol.
- Drink plenty of water to replace losses through perspiration, listen to your body, watch for signals of over-exertion.

It is Never too Late to Take the Crucial First Step Towards Fitness

- Anxiety and stress can affect the heart.
- What is depression?
- Stress is an unavoidable fact of life. Some stresses are part of daily life. It affects everyone.
- An old proverb cautions us that 'the brain may hold a conversation with the heart that can result in death'
- Are some people more prone to stress?
- What causes stress?
- This could be personal loss, death of a loved one, separation, divorce. Change of job, money problem, debts, loss of steady income, illness, change in family structure, retirement, etc.

What are Early Warning Signs of Stress?

- Constant feeling of exhaustion.
- Frequent illness, including headaches, insomnia, indigestion, nausea, diarrhea, constipation.

- Excessive worrying about.
- Mental fatigue, difficulty in concentrating.
- Irritability, sense of worthlessness.
- Personal neglect.
- Stay positive, learn to relax, get as much sleep as you need.
- It is not always possible to avoid stress but one has to change towards life through spiritual practices such as meditation and yoga.

Remember that life is 10% what happens to you and 90% how you react to it, be optimistic. It helps being realistic, planning your work, taking a break, learning to relax.

Medicines: If our cholesterol level is very high and not reduced with diet and exercise, then drug may be necessary. Continue with diet and exercise therapy.

REGULAR DRUG TO CONTROL BLOOD PRESSURE

Why do People Smoke?

The reasons are several: Nicotinic craving—it is a powerful stimulant, which is harmful to the heart. In addition, the substance causes the dependence on cigarettes.

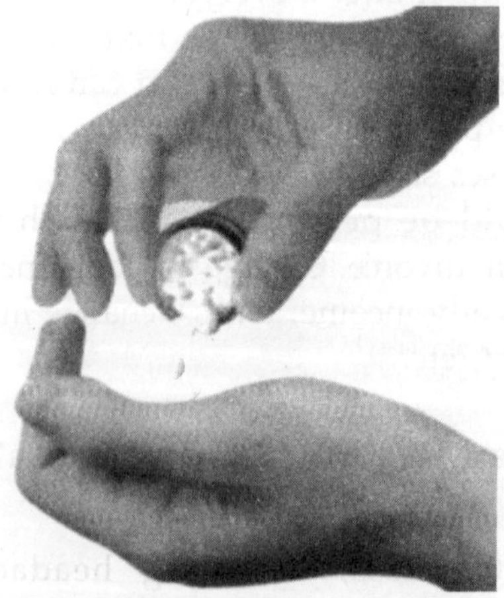

Fig. 1.7: Drug to control blood pressure

This is evident if you need to have a cigarette within 30 minutes of awakening in the morning, or feel irritable and have a headache after a movie or a long meeting in which you could not smoke, habit smoking, e.g. in the toilet, driving to work, etc.

Carbon monoxide is a poisonous gas which decreases the efficiency of the heart and lungs to deliver oxygen to the tissues. Tar—which is full of cancer-causing chemicals.

Mood smoking when you are depressed, bored, relaxing. etc. Social smoking because others in your group are smoking. Smokers have twice the risk of having heart attacks as non-smokers. Smoking causes stroke, high blood pressure, circulation of lungs, lung cancer, and affects general well-being. Smoking is a social evil. It gives bad breath and stains teeth. You have irritating cough, food tastes bad, you spend more money, and cuts lifespan.

Cutting down on cigarettes will result in more oxygen supply to your brain and increases concentration.

Enjoyment is short-lived, you feel you are getting relaxed, but it raises your blood pressure. Decide positively that you want to quit. Be confident about your ability to stop. You have more will power than you think.

Avoid myths, as I do not have the will power to quit. Quit once, I can stop whenever I want, but I want to enjoy it for some more time. I felt terrible the last time, I quit. I have smoked for so long, I am sure the damage is already done. I can stop later, there is no hurry. All my friends smoke. Why worry? Everybody is going to die when their time comes.

- Stop carrying cigarettes with you.
- Limit the places and circumstances where you smoke.
- Change the situation in which you smoke.
- Change the way you smoke.
- Concentrate each cigarette you smoke.
- Keep a smoking diary.
- Advertise your near ones for your quitting.
- Decide how to reward yourself for quitting.
- Throw all cigarettes, matches, ashtrays.

- Visit dentist and have your teeth cleaned of tobacco stains.
- Keep yourself busy, go to movies, exercise, take a long walk, go bike riding.
- Reach for a glass of juice instead of a cigarette.
- Start thinking of yourself as a nonsmoker.

HIGH BLOOD PRESSURE IS A SILENT KILLER

Sphygmomanometer Used to Detect Blood Pressure

What is Blood Pressure?

Systolic pressure reading between 120 and 130 and a diastolic pressure reading between 80 and 90.

- The diastolic pressure be maintained below 90 if possible.
- Your blood pressure tells your doctor a great deal about your health.
- Low blood pressure is far less common than hypertension.

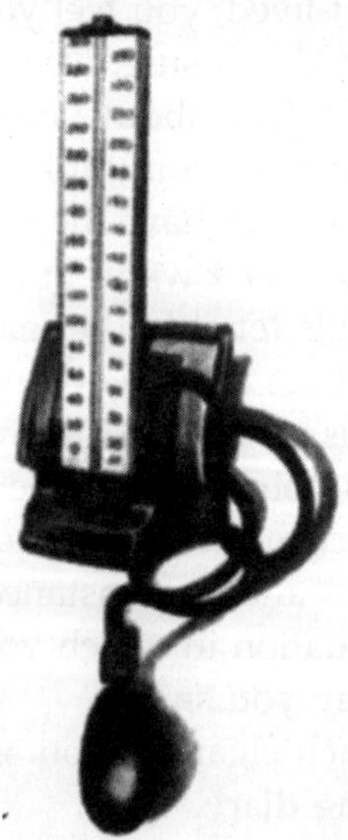

Fig. 1.8: Sphygmomanometer

- High blood pressure is a very common condition seen in modern life. However, in great majority of cases we are still at a loss to explain why the pressure is elevated. We can measure the rising pressure. But why does it start to rise? This is still a mystery.
- Why we are concerned about high blood pressure/if left untreated, what can hypertension do?

HYPERTENSION CAN AFFECT YOUR HEART

When there is a coronary blockage, which cannot be treated by drugs—Bypass Surgery Indicated

Heart—Leading to angina, heart attack, or lead to enlarged heart, which cannot work efficiently and may ultimately end up as congestive heart failure with water accumulation in the lungs.

Brain—Continuous high blood pressure on the arteries of the brain may lead to a blood clot or ruptured artery in the brain. Loss of memory, blindness, speech difficulty or paralysis may follow.

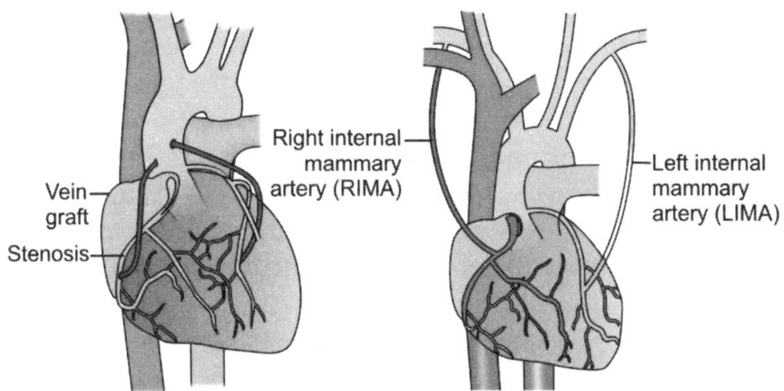

Fig. 1.9: Bypass surgery and life after bypass surgery

Kidneys—Persistently high blood pressure will damage the delicate filtering units of the kidney. This can result in uremia, swelling of the body and kidney failure, necessitating dialysis or kidney transplantation.

Eyes—As a result of the high blood pressure, walls of the blood vessels in the eyes thicken. This leads to deterioration of vision, possibility of bleeding into the eyes and ultimately blindness.

What Causes Hypertension?

- In most cases the cause of hypertension remains unknown
- Heredity—It runs in family
- Age—Older people more likely to have than younger
- Stress—Anxiety, competitiveness and hostility may increase
- Excessive sodium
- Overweight.

Drugs

- What is secondary high blood pressure (HBP)?
- How can it be detected?
- What good does treatment do?
- What leads people to default their treatment?
- How you can control your HBP?
- How can family and friends help in controlling HBP?
- Does BP increase with age?
- Can children have HBP?
- Is medication need to be taken for lifelong?

Never discontinue, decrease or substitute medication without consulting your physician. This can result in dangerous changes in blood pressure. Establish daily routine, report side effects, maintain BP chart, keep all appointment with cardiologist.

In what other way conclusion–
- Medical management
- Lifestyle modification
- Weight reduction

- Sodium restriction
- Dietary modification
- Exercise
- Alcohol restriction
- Caffeine restriction
- Relaxation technique
- Smoking cessation
- Potassium supplementation
- Pharmacologic intervention
- Beta-blockers
- Vasodilators
- Calcium antagonist
- Angiogenin converting enzyme
- Nursing management.

DIAGNOSIS AND INVESTIGATIONS FOR HEART DISEASES

- Electrocardiography
- Echocardiography
- Coronary angiography and angioplasty
- Bypass surgery
- Stress testing
- Coronary stent
- Blood cholesterol.

An Incentive Spirometer from Which You will Require Sucking Sufficiently, Hard to Keep Plastic Balls Floating in the Air

How can I Lower My Blood Pressure?

Lose weight, exercise, reduce salt intake, reduce alcohol intake, reduce stress, stop smoking.

Remember

1. High blood pressure can be controlled and not cured just like diabetes.

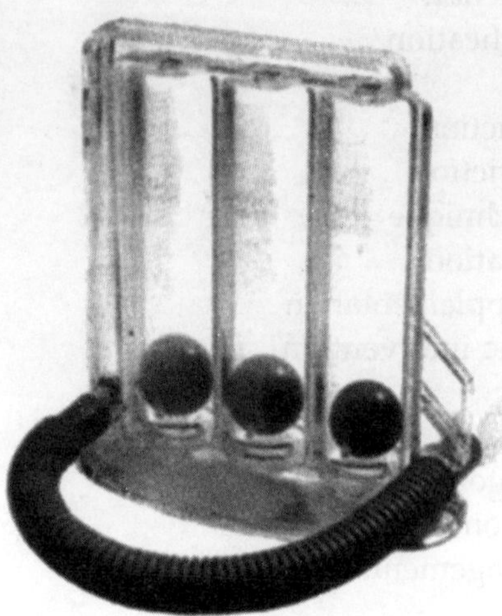

Fig. 1.10: An incentive spirometer

2. Have your blood pressure checked regularly and follow your physicians advice.
3. Your blood pressure will remain normal just as long as you take your medicines.
4. In general, medicines will need to be taken lifelong.
5. Some minor inconveniences of taking medicines will greatly improve your ultimate quantity and quality of life.
6. If you do all these, you can feel better and live longer. So do them now. You deserve to be healthy for as long as you live.

Exhibition Value of Project

After the detailed study ourselves, we improved our knowledge regarding cardiovascular disease and understood as a nurse how important it is to save life of people entrusted in our hands. We understood the preciousness of life and the importance of taking its good care.

• It added developed confidence how to face the crowd and how to talk in public.

- We also could see with our own eyes the positive feedback and the outcome.
- We also learnt to be creative and from least expense, we can give the maximum.
- Learnt effective health education method.
- We brought smile on people's face and our excellent report to the teacher.
- It was a great and newer experience.
- Overall project was economical.
- Community benefited.
- We were satisfied with the outcome.

2 | # Model Exhibition Project on Balanced Diet

BALANCE DIET

Introduction

This is a project on "Balanced Diet" which deals with the full nutritional status of the people.

We have taken this topic to teach the group of people about the balanced diet and make them understand about what diet they should take to prevent nutritional diseases. The dietary pattern varies widely in different parts of the world.

Balanced diet is a kind of food on which a person or group lives. It contains a variety of foods in such a quantities and proportions that the need for energy, amino acid, vitamins, minerals, fats, carbohydrates and other nutrients is adequately met for maintaining health, vitality and generally withstand short duration of leanness. Recommended daily intake is nutrient sufficient for the maintenance of health in nearly all people. There is optimum requirement, minimum requirement, and safe level of intake.

Definition

A balanced diet is defined as one, which provides:
1. A sufficient number of calories.
2. An adequate amount of protein, fat and carbohydrate.
3. An adequate amount of vitamins and minerals for maintaining health, vitality and general well-being.

Composition of Balanced Diet (Fig. 2.1)

If the diet is inadequate in one or some of the below elements, malnutrition may occur and the human body becomes physically and mentally hampered. The vitality is lowered, and a person has a low capacity to work.

Cereals	-	400 gm
Pulses	-	55 to 70 gm
Leafy vegetables	-	100 gm
Other vegetables	-	75 gm
Roots and tubers	-	5 gm
Milk	-	200 gm
Fats	-	30 gm
Meat/fish	-	30 gm
Egg	-	30 gm
Fruits	-	30 gm
Sugar	-	30 gm

BALANCED DIET PROVIDES A SUFFICIENT NUMBER OF CALORIES

Recommended Daily Allowances of Calories

1. Man 55 kg—work sedentary net calories 2400; moderate 2800 and heavy 3900 calories
2. Woman 45 kg—sedentary 2000; moderate 2300; heavy 3000; pregnancy 2300; lactation 2700 calories
3. Children 0 to 6 months 120/kg
4. Adolescents 13 to 15 year old girls 2100; boys 2500
5. Adolescents 16 to 19 year old girls 2100; boys 3150 calories.

Members of the Group

1.
2.
3.
4
5
6.

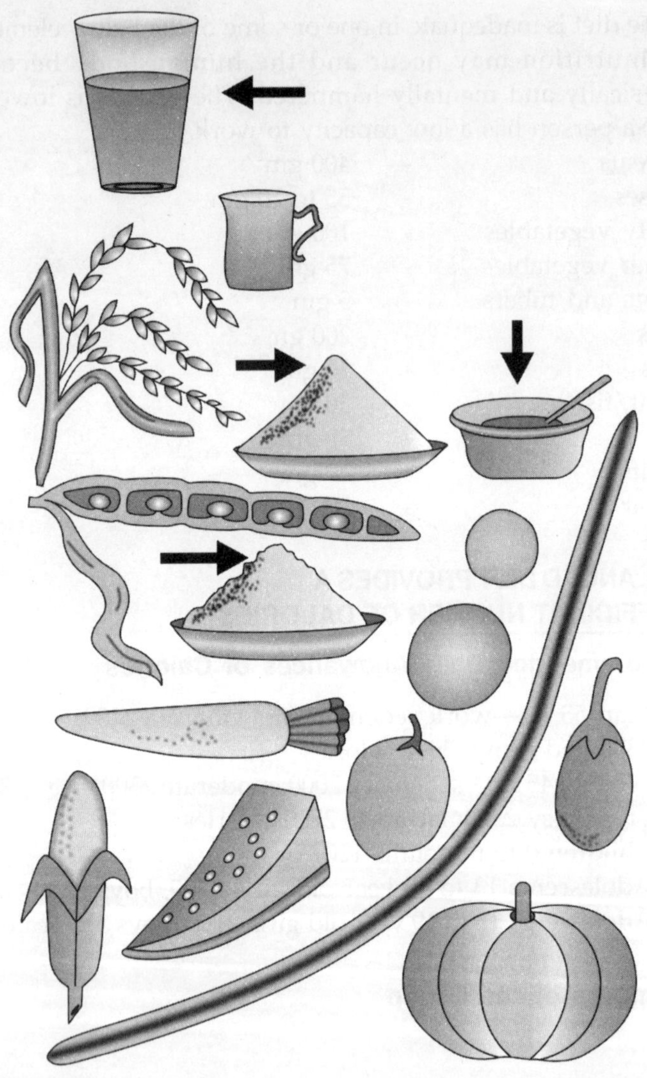

Fig. 2.1: Balanced diet

Title of the Project: Balanced Diet

1. Form of project: Group
2. Type of project: Portable and could shift easily and carry from institution to the field area
3. Name of the institution
4. Year of study
5. Name of the groups:
   i.
   ii.
   iii.
   iv.
   v.
   vi.

Date of Commencement

1. Date of completion of project
2. Name of the teacher submitted.

Need of the Project

- To educate the people about malnutritional diseases occurring due to lack of nutritional diet.
- Protein-energy malnutrition, endemic goiter, nutritional anemia, nutritional blindness and diarrheal disease.
- The association of nutrition with infection, immunity, fertility.
- Low birth weight is a major public health problem.
- Food-borne infections, e.g. typhoid, food poisoning, *E. coli*, etc. Food-borne diseases are usually either infectious or toxic in nature, caused by agents that enter the body through the ingestion of food.
- Nutrition is the cornerstone of socioeconomic development and its problems are not just medical but are multifactor.
- To educate the people about the vegetables, pulses, fruits etc., and what are their contents.

- To educate people to handle food, utensils, dish wash, sanitation of eating places, place of meal served and to develop clean habits.

Planning of the Project

The group members have prepared song on the "Balanced Diet" topic and prepared skit, showing different types of diseases, occurring due to lack of nutrition. We had prepared flash cards and on the white cloth we distributed the pulses, vegetables, fruits, meat, fish, milk. We had planned to dance with all the vegetables. We decided to explain every topic by each person of the group by turns.

Background Information of Area

A small village situated in Thane district named Usgaon, consisting of 250 families. The houses build over here are both *kachcha* and *pucca* houses. *Anganwadi* and primary school are situated in this area. It has also a market and general stores. No sanitary latrines are available to the people in there homes. There is a river passing by which has water all through year. Therefore, we decided to take up this topic so at least they can have kitchen garden and cultivate some green vegetables. When planning balanced diet, it is important to know what foods are available according to origin, an intake of different types of foods desired to archieve optimum health.

Survey

According to the plan, we had conducted a survey in Usgaon and we came to know that there are approximately 200-250 families residing in this area. According to survey, PHC has been located in the main center and there are different subcenters in this area. If any problem persists in any family, they are transferred to PHC. In PHC there are immunization program, antenatal clinics held as per different days while OPD is functioning during the day for minor ailments, treatment and deliveries conducted. While doing the survey of different families visited, we came to conclusion that the members of many different families are affected with different nutritional diseases mainly malnutrition and anemia. There is a poor maintenance of personal hygiene and poor environmental sanitation.

Goals and Objectives

1. To give the information about preventing the nutritional disease.
2. To reach out to the people to give knowledge about nutrition.
3. To prevent nutritional disease.
4. To give out various information through various audiovisual aids such as charts, flash cards, flannel board and models, etc.
5. To build energy and strengthen muscles and bones.
6. To repair tissue.
7. To give knowledge to the people how to make nutritional balance by home-made things.
8. To demonstrate how locally available food be converted into nutritious diet.
9. Explain the difference of foods of animal origin and foods of vegetable origin.
10. Explain foods that build body, foods that give energy, foods that protect body.

Assessment of Resources

We, as a team, (Fig. 2.2) decided to start our exhibition by explaining different kinds of fruits, pulses with the flash cards, posters and flannel board.

We had prepared kitchen orchestra, where we explained the diet, treatment and prevention.

We had a skit and jagruti theme songs and slogans prepared explaining all the important nutritional diseases.

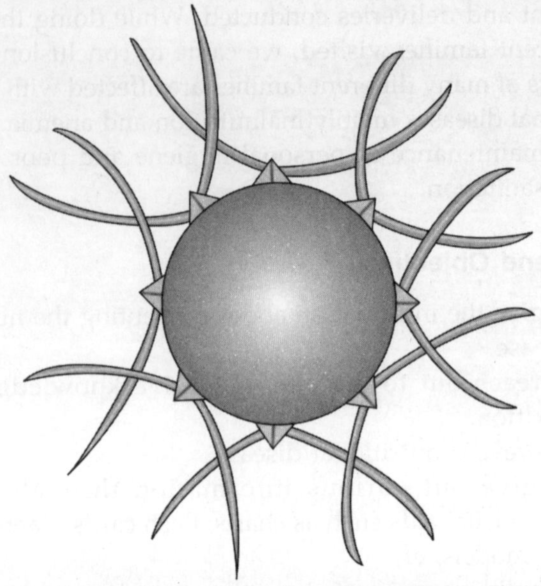

Fig. 2.2: Working together for health

Equipment Required

Resources available—Chart paper, cardboards, sketch pens, water color, brown paper, sparkle colors, different types of pulses, vegetables and fruits, CD player, table, chair, artificial house with garden, bed sheet, clay, locally available things like stone, mud, sticks, etc.

Manpower/Work Force Required

1.
2.
3.
4.
5.
6.

Appropriate Technology

Demonstration, variable explanation with skit and songs and dance, local language.
Organization
Workplace—rural area of posting.

Schedule of Stages Start to Finish Time

* 4.00 pm (Fig. 2.3), reached at the spot and displayed all the charts and posters.
* 4.30 to 5.00 pm, arranged all the articles.
* 5.00 to 5.30 pm, went to the village and invited once again the people for the same.
* 5.30 to 7 pm, explained about the definition, sources, prevention and treatment of the diseases and the importance of balanced diet.
* 7 to 7.30 pm, gave small refreshment to the people and children gathered and ended the program with a jagruti song and made people to repeat the slogans.

Controlling

Allocated Responsibility to Each Members

1. Explanation of all the fruits and thier contents and their deficiency results.
2. Explanation of all the vegetables and their content and lack of them causes in what.
3. Explanation of pulses and what they get from them and how they affect if not taken in a balanced way in our diet.
4. Explanation of meat, fish, milk and eggs and lack of it causes in what.
5. Explanation of variations done by specifying protein and its functions and its deficiency.
6. Explain fat, calcium, minerals and vitamins.
7. How one can prevent the diseases.

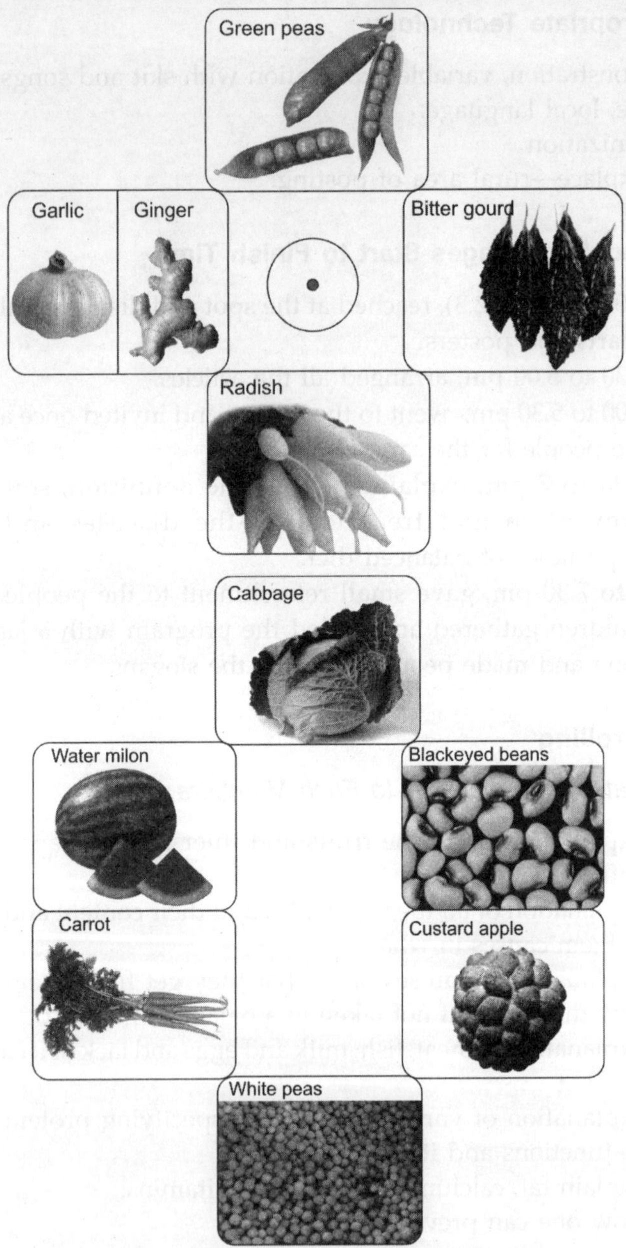

Fig. 2.3: Charts and posters

Fixing of Priority

As we went into the field, surveyed, and visited people in their homes, balwadies, schools, etc. We found that nutritional diseases were affected to many people. One thing we found they were poor socially and economically yet they had some foods, vegetables of the seasons, they were not having. They had fixed kind of routine diet, which was insufficient, not nutritious and lacked in vital vitamins. Due to prolonged lack of it, they had developed certain pigmentation diseases, anemia, etc. So we gave our top priority to this topic. In addition, fixed priority as a team to take up balanced diet.

- We gathered people for the exhibition of our project and we had preplanned aims and objectives.
- We started in time as we had already informed people by going to door-to-door visit before the program and invited them to come for the same.
- We began with a song and welcomed the people.
- We introduced the group and the topic.
- Then we went to the topic explaining and showing them the different aids, we had prepared, the importance of healthy diet, nutrient, the source of nutrition, etc.
- Explained how malnutrition can be prevented. What is the difference between who had nutritious food and those who did not have by comparing posters.
- We played a skit and role-play showing how we can prevent nightblindness by taking this diet.
- How we can prevent calcium deficiency, anemia, kwashiorkor and marasmus.
- Through jagruti songs and slogans, we gave information about food hygiene.
- We guided them how they can get these food in and around the village which are seasonal and not costly.
- Helped them to see the value of kitchen garden.

Collection of Data

- Books, newspapers, magazines, family services, internet, teacher's help.
- We tried to use the data according to the needs of the people and the types of group we had with us. We demonstrated and even made the children to understand how to have healthy foods that are available in their own fields.

Implementation

Classroom knowledge and people's lifestyle we build the topic and reached to them in their own style.

Overall Project

Satisfying and happy with outcome.

Benefit of Community

As we had, variation in our approach people did not feel bored and were enthusiastic and attentive and found interested to know more. By displaying this exhibition, they came to know the importance of healthy balanced diet and its advantages and disadvantages. They understood how certain diseases come due to imbalance of it. We had living models to show this deficiency. Now what to add to the diet they understood and eager to try out. We found the feeling of convictions on their faces.

Educational Value of Project

After the detail study in our preplanning, we too improved our knowledge and understanding and our role and function as a nurse to promote healthy balanced diet and teach the people who come in our contact. Though we knew some things yet after this project, we too were enlightened, motivated, and became aware of it in a renewed way thus our will was strengthened.

INNOVATIVE APPROACH AND GROUP PRESENTATION

United We Stand Divided We Fall

As we had given health talks on similar topics but all the audiovisual aids combined with team spirit, it was a wonderful experience for us and people as well. We could see the fruit of our efforts when people clapped and said words of encouragements.

Subject Matter

What is a Balanced Diet?

A balanced diet is defined as a provider of a sufficient number of calories, adequate amount of vitamins and minerals for maintaining health, vitality and general well-being.

VEGETABLES

Adequate Amount of Protein, Fat and Carbohydrate

Experts in nutrition have classified vegetables into three groups.

Green Leafy Vegetables

There is a wide variety of green leafy vegetables. Palak, amaranth sour green, cabbage, methis, etc. They are the cheapest among "protective foods." Green leafy vegetables are valuable from the point of human nutrition. They are excellent and inexpensive sources of carotene, B-group vitamins and minerals. They contain cellulose, which acts as "roughage" in the intestine, and helps prevent constipation.

Roots and Tubers

The common vegetables in this group are potatoes, tapioca, carrot, onion, etc. Potatoes and tapioca contain plenty of starch. Carrot is rich in carotene. In general, roots and tubers are

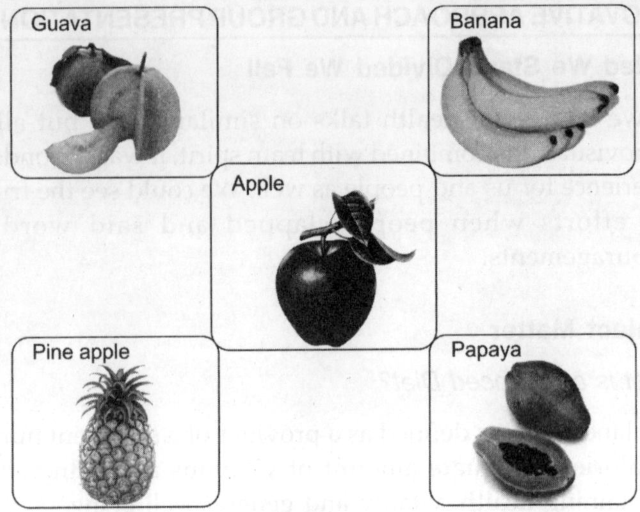

Fig. 2.4: Fruits

good sources of minerals such as calcium and potassium and vitamins and carbohydrate too.

Other Vegetables

All the remaining vegetables, e.g. brinjals, tomatoes, cauliflowers are considered in this group. They too contain good source of vitamins, iron, etc.

FRUITS (FIG. 2.4)

Fruits give strength, stamina and build immunity in preserving your life and are protective foods. They are invaluable in human nutrition. They can be eaten fresh and raw. This makes the vitamins present in fruits easily available. *Nutritive value*–fruits are prized for vitamins especially vitamin C and carotene. The common papaya and mango are good rich sources of minerals and sulphur. Some fruits like sitaphal are rich in calcium. Therefore, each fruit has its unique quality.

PULSES (FIG. 2.5)

An Adequate Amount of Vitamins and Minerals for Maintaining Health, Vitality and General Well-Being

Pulses are the best known like red gram, green gram, black gram, Bengal gram/chana. They are rich sources of protein. They are called poor man's meat because they are the main sources of protein for the poor man's diet. They are also good sources of B-group vitamins and minerals. Germinating pulses contain vitamin C.

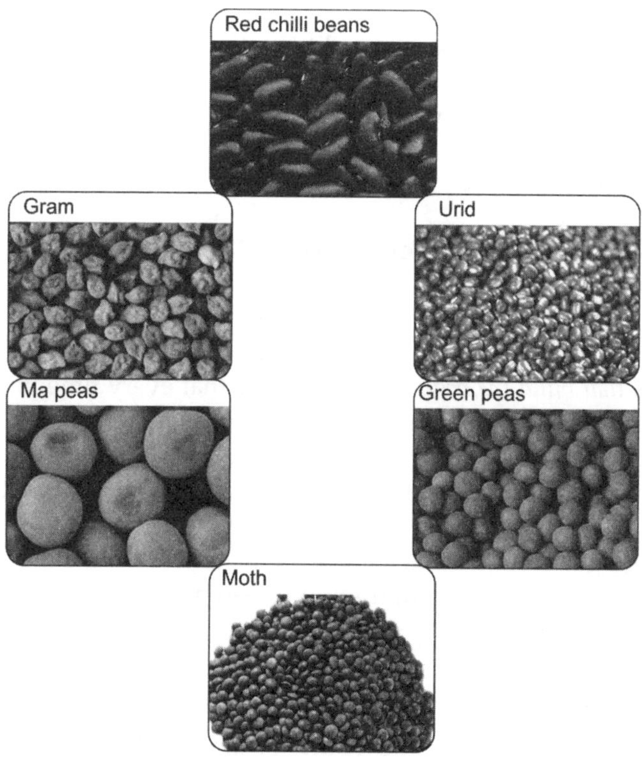

Fig. 2.5: Pulses

ANIMAL FOOD

Meat—The term meat refers to the flesh of cattle, sheep and pigs. Meat contains 20% proteins. Meat is rich in iron and phosphorus.

Fish Has Many Varieties Both Fresh and Salted

Sweet water fish and salt water fish. The composition of fish is given as protein 21.5 gm; 1.6 gm fat, 2.0 minerals. Fish is good source of calcium and phosphorus. Sea fish contains iodine.

Eggs—Contain all the food factors except carbohydrates. The white of the egg amount to about 60%, the yolk about 30% and the outer shell 10%. Therefore, ducks egg should not be eaten raw.

We explained the disease conditions through a skit (Fig. 2.6).

- Kwashiorkor and marasmus.
- Calcium deficiency.
- Anemia.
- Night blindness.

Lack of Calcium in Diet Leads to Calcium Deficiency Disease

Subject Matter

Foods that build the body–did you know that every time you sit down to a meal, you make an important decision concerning your own future. What you and how you eat it may determine how long you live, and whether you will be sick or well. If you lack balanced diet, you will be neither sick nor well just dragging around, half-dead most of the time. What a miserable existence. Not sick enough to go to bed and not well enough to work properly.

What are the Principles of Good Living?

All forms of life, whether plants or animals, require certain essential food elements in order to live and reproduce their

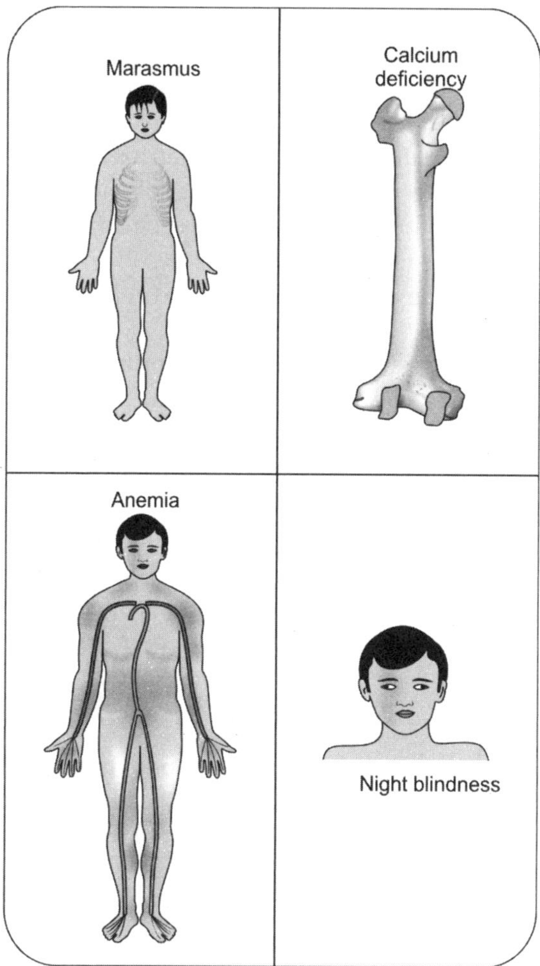

Fig. 2.6: Different deficiency diseases

own kind. These food materials must be present in the diet in the right proportion, and must be taken regularly.

Human body is composed of untold millions of living cells whose function each cell must be fed and cared for or else they will not work properly. To have sensible diet is an important decision. It depends on our right choice of food.

The human body has been beautifully engineered, provided we treat it well. The body has a power to combat illness, fight disease, and replace worn-out tissue with new living cells.

Good building materials essential—when a man plans to build a house, he first secures the best materials he can afford. He tries to order just the right amount of each so there will be no waste. Then he begins to build.

The same is true of this most wonderful house, our human body.

- What are these bodybuilding materials: Proteins, fats, carbohydrates, vitamins, minerals and water?
- Why proteins are so important in the diet?
- Why is the body so dependent on protein?

If you touch a piece of metal on a cool day, it feels cold and hard. But the skin of your face feels soft and warm. Why? Because that skin is pulsating with life. The metal is cold and lifeless. Skin is composed with living cells, untold myriads of them, each with its special function to perform.

What has all this to do with food?

What you eat keeps the cell alive. Body is build from the proteins within our diet. Proteins are needed continually to repair worn-out tissues. They are essential for building strong bones and muscles.

Richest sources of protein are whole-grain cereals, peas, beans, lentils, peanuts, soybeans, milk, eggs, cheese, butter milk, meat and fish.

Where do we find them in our daily diet?

Vitamins and minerals entirely come from plants and animals foods. We cannot live very long with imbalanced diet. So in planning food purchases, try to provide the best-balanced meals.

The minerals in your body have many important functions to perform. Calcium and phosphorus are needed for building strong bones and teeth. Without these, the body would quickly collapse. Calcium found in the bones where it provides strength and stability to the whole system. It helps to prevent hemorrhage. Lack of it, muscles go into spasm, cramping pain; it helps irregular beating of the heart. Lack of it can cause rickets in children, he suffers marked weakness in the bones, considered delay in sitting up, crawling, and walking, joint out of shape they bent, causing deformities as bow-legs, pigeon breast, and knock knees. In addition, osteomalacia in adult where bones flattened and pelvic outlet narrowed, spinal bone shortens, and individual looses height and becomes dwarfed and stooped. However, the individual must also have sufficient sunshine to derive benefit of vitamin D and calcium in the diet.

Source of calcium is milk, dairy products, green vegetables, peas, beans, soybeans, eggs, lentils, potatoes, and fish. In other words, well-balanced diet usually has sufficient calcium to meet our needs.

Another important mineral is iron. Most of the iron is found in the red blood cells, where it forms part of that very complex protein known as hemoglobin. This is the substance that gives color to the blood. It carries oxygen to the tissues and keeps us alive.

Source—many foods contain iron but all of it is not absorbed. Green leaves, eggs, apricots, raisins, potatoes, liver, etc. are all good sources of iron.

Preserving minerals—when preparing food, do not loose it with carelessness. Important nutrients thrown with the water.

Nature makes no mistakes in preparing food. What was this secret substance in fruits and vegetables that prevent scurvy?

Vitamin A is the beauty vitamin. It helps to keep the skin smooth and soft. It is also needed for the mucous membranes lining the nose, throat, digestive tract, the bladder, etc. It aids in the normal growth of bones and teeth.

When people are healthy and strong, extra vitamins are not needed. They are valuable when a person is recovering from severe illness or injury. Most people can get all the vitamins they need by taking a well-balanced diet, along with sufficient rest, sunshine and exercise.

Proteins constitute about 20% of the body weight in an adult. Man derives protein from a variety of food sources. People must eat mixed diet. When planning balanced diet, it is important to know what foods are available according to origin, an intake of different types of foods is desired to achieve good health.

Fruits are prized for their vitamins. Most fruits contain significant amounts of ascorbic acid, fruits contain cellulose which assists in normal bowel movements. Fruits are costly and it may not be within the reach of all to afford them daily. Seasonal fruits are cheaper and easily available if leafy vegetables are included in diet need for fruits is reduced.

Action at the Family Level

1. Education on the selection of right kind of local foods and nutritionally adequate diets within the limits of their purchasing power.
2. Harmful food taboos and dietary prejudices can be identified and corrected to promote breastfeeding.
3. Planning of kitchen garden and keeping poultry.
4. Regular health checkups.
5. Increasing agricultural production.
6. The family plays an important role in shaping the food habits which are passed from generation to generation.
7. Starvation in the midst of plenty, people choose poor diets when good ones available because of cultural influences, customs, beliefs, traditions and attitudes.
8. Cooking practices like draining away the rice water at the end of cooking, prolonged boiling in open pans, peeling of vegetables all influence the nutritive value of food.
9. By product of poverty, ignorance, insufficient education, lack of knowledge regarding nutritive values of food.
10. Nutritional surveillances and growth monitoring.

11. Nurses have a responsibility of teaching good nutrition to remove prejudices and impart good dietary habits. Practically, doing cooking demonstration, exhibition and kitchen gardening and practical methods of education.

It is said that there will be very little malnutrition in India today if all the food available can be equitably distributed in accordance with physiological needs.

Gave Awareness of Community Nutritional Program

The Government of India has initiated several large-scale supplementary feeding programs, and programs aimed at overcoming specific deficiency diseases through various ministries to combat malnutrition, e.g. ICDS program, mid-day meal program, balwadi nutrition, etc.

We ended the program by a kitchen group dance with all the vegetables and fruits.

Gave all the people gathered, one banana each while explained the following:

Note—Amazing Fruit—Bananas

Never put bananas in the refrigerator. Banana contains natural sugars, sucrose, fructose and glucose combined with fiber, and vitamin B_6. It gives an instant, sustained and substantial boost of energy. Research has proven that just two bananas provide enough energy for strenuous 90-minute workouts and overcome a number of illness. You must add it to your diet. Unique tropical fruit, low in salt, making it perfect to beat BP, makes students more alert, overcomes constipation, heartburn, morning sickness, nerves, ulcers, temperature control, stress, strokes, warts, etc. It is a natural remedy for many ills.

Keep General Principles of Cooking

1. Fresh vegetables contain more vitamin C than stored ones.
2. Vegetables must be checked for mold and worm infection, salad vegetables must be fresh, firm and crisp.

3. Tomatoes must be examined for mold, spoilage around the stalk.
4. Over-riped fruits should not be purchased.
5. All food grains should be kept in dry, clean and airtight tins.
6. Cut vegetables just before cooking, do not cut in very small pieces, cook in slow fire, do not use baking soda as it destroys vitamin content.
7. Prolonged cooking destroys vitamins.
8. Excessive water after cooking use in dals.
9. Do not keep cooked food exposed, refrigerated foods should be reheated before consumption.
10. Salad should be prepared just before serving.

Methods of cooking—boiling, simmering, steaming, frying, roasting, baking.

Methods of food preservation—drying, cold storage, smoking, pickling, addition of sugar, freezing, chemical preservation, etc.

Model Project Exhibition on Environmental Sanitation

1. Do not defecate in open air (Fig. 3.1).

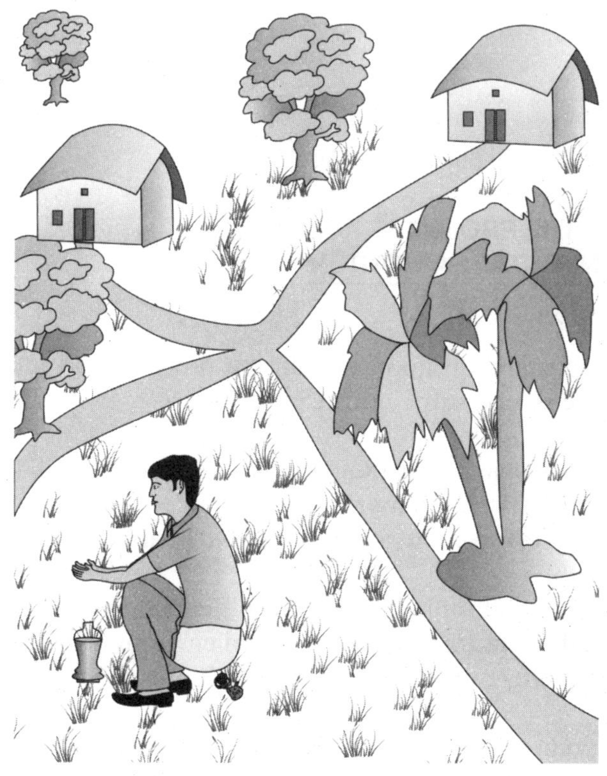

Fig. 3.1: A person defecating in open air

2. Do not use contaminated water for drinking (Fig. 3.2).

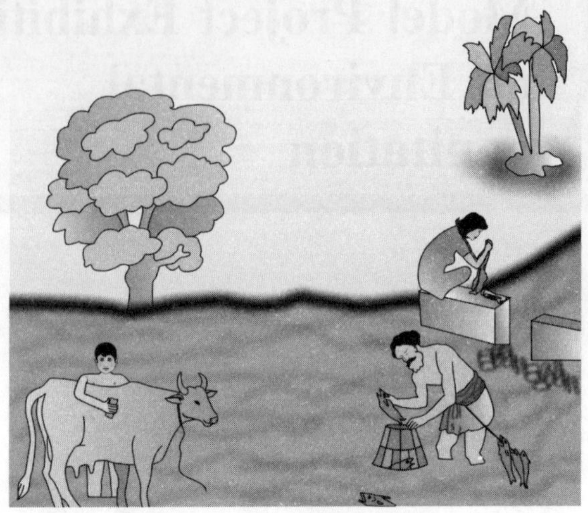

Fig. 3.2: Contaminated water

TITLE OF THE PROJECT–
ENVIRONMENTAL SANITATION

Introduction

In order to maintain good health, the physical and mental health care is not sufficient, it is necessary to take care of surrounding hygiene.

Human beings are surrounded by air, water and soil; these together comprise his environment along with other living beings. Therefore, the key to man's health lies in his environment.

Environmental sanitation has been defined by WHO "the control of these factor in man's physical environment which a deleterious effect on his physical development, health and survival".

Environment also affects the social and economic condition under which man is surrounded that is his customs, culture and habits.

To safeguard man's health the control of all these factors are important component of community health, because much of ill health is due to unsafe water, polluted soil and unhygienic disposal of human excreta (Fig. 3.1).

Human excreta are the source of infection. It contains pathogenic bacteria, protozoa, helminthes parasites and their eggs.

Therefore, it must be disposed of in a hygienic manner.

Statistics indicate more than 50 million people in India suffer from worm infestation.

Therefore, it is the responsibility of community worker to educate people about hygiene and improvement of sanitation to prevent disease. To educate people and to get cooperation from them we have prepared this exhibition project.

We have taken this topic to teach people in rural areas about proper sanitation and make them understand the techniques of taking care of nature gifted by God.

The dictionary meaning of the word sanitation of "the science of safeguarding health".

Definition—sanitation is a way of life, it is the quality of living that is expressed in the clean home, the clean farm, the clean business, the clean neighborhood and clean community.

Planning of the Project Exhibition

As a group went out into the field and as we went around investigating and visiting families in the area we observed unhygienic condition, which had effects on people's health and their living. This motivated the group to take up the challenge of preparing project form exhibition.

The exhibition was planned out to educate and impart knowledge regarding environmental sanitation and cleanliness.

The project dealt with the correct manner of disposing waste, planting of trees, cleanliness of wells, etc.

Preplan

* To match the limited resources at hand.

- To eliminate wasteful expenditure.
- To develop best course of action.
- To accomplish defined objectives.

We preplanned our purpose focusing on the rescores at hand working as a team taking the things around in the nature low cost.

Background Information of the Area

We planned to conduct our exhibition in PHC since it was a ANC clinic day besides a routine OPD. We could get good number of people from close by villages that we had visited. Thus, this enhanced us to put forward our views and ideas through this project effectively.

Survey if Any

We had a complete survey of the area as we had one-month posting in the field we could cover up the entire given areas. We found during our visits that there was lack of proper sanitation (Fig. 3.2), open-air defecation (Fig. 3.1), and there was no proper disposal of waste.

Therefore, after conducting survey and data collection we priories on this point environmental hygiene. In addition, put up on the same topic with the cooperation and help of the local villagers living in the community.

Goals

- To maintain personal hygiene and keep the surrounding clean.
- To motivate the people to maintain proper environmental hygiene.
- To decline the number of health problems arising due to poor sanitation.
- To help the people realize the disadvantages and bad effect of open air defecation.

- To impart the people with adequate knowledge regarding proper refuse disposal.

Objectives

- To make group understand the meaning of environmental hygiene.
- The group is able to list down the importance of environmental health.
- To explain about the different components.
- To explain about the methods of refuse disposal and its bad effect on health.
- To make the target group understand the preventive and promotive measures.

Assessment of Resources

Such as work force, money/budget, materials available, skills, creativity, talents, knowledge, technique, time needed all these directed towards objectives.

The resources used towards were cheap and affordable, easily available and cost effective and economical low cost type that were naturally available like grass, plants, mud, stones, tharmocoal and so on.

The resources used were very effective, e.g. mud we used to make a well and dustbin, sticks were used to make broom and cowshed, various drainage were drawn on chart papers to show the real environmental sanitation.

Fixing of Priority

The priority we selected was as follows:
1. To sweep the surrounding as well as the house twice daily.
2. To avoid open air defecation.
3. To avoid washing clothes in the same river or around the well where the water is used for drinking purpose.
4. Proper disposal of garbage like dumping, composting, etc.

5. Well should be covered with net and away from sewage.
6. Cleaning and bathing of animals separately and that water should drain under the ground.
7. Cowshed should be clean and not in the house itself if possible.
8. Maintain personal and community hygiene to prevent diseases, e.g. worm infestation.

Expected Outcome of the Project

- We expected that people understand about proper environmental sanitation.
- Trees should not be cut.
- Community toilets should be used and open air defecation should be avoided.
- Proper disposal of excreta should be done.
- Total eradication of diseases that occurs due to lack of sanitation, which could be prevented by joint effort.
- Environmental sanitation.
- Maintenance of personal and community hygiene.
- Preventing mode of transmission of worm infestation.
- To give the village a clean tidy face.
- To have more shady trees.
- Each one takes this as an personal commitment.
- Teaching and developing cultivating these habits in young children who can follow elders as a role model and see values in it.
- The other surrounding other villages too follows and knows the benefits of environmental sanitation in there personal and village life.
- Regular evaluation of the progress and its achievements.

Implementation

We implemented project as we had preplanned systematically and gradually step by step. Used the resources that were available such as thermocol, pins, chart papers, gum, Fevicol, sketch pen, water colors, grass, leaves, sticks, cardboard, etc

Work Force Required

- Seven members shared the responsibilities as preplanned assignments to avoid confusion and duplication, this save time and be effective.
  - Introduction to the topic selected.
  - Explained about the health hazards that occur due to lack of sanitation.
- Explain the meaning of open-air defecation and effects on health.
- Explained about the garbage and its ill effect on health when not disposed in proper way.
- Drawing, carving of thermocol, preparation of charts, painting, fixing, arrangements, and over all management
- Last one concluded and summarize with feedback.

Equipment Required

- An open space where people could gather and have view so had big tables and chairs.
- Cot, strings, and all the above-mentioned things.

Appropriate Technology

- Based on scientific and nursing principles.
- Practical demonstration with educational charts and discussion.
- Each group member took active part, which was correlated with scientifically principles.
- What we learnt in classroom, and what we observed in actual field based on it we build the simple techniques which was understood by simple people.

SCHEDULE OF STAGES START TO FINISH USED PROPERLY

Definition

- Explanation of clean environment.
- Explanation of unclean surrounding.

- Difference of clean and unclean.
- Prevention of disease occur due to lack of it.
- Methods of garbage disposal.
- Ill effects of washing clothes or bathing animals in the same river from where water is consumed.
- The group showed cooperation, interest and team spirit.
- Build rapport, communication skill, presentation skill, hard work, and set goals were satisfactorily achieved.
- All the members participated creatively with enthusiasm working hard for the cause towards completion of the project.

Controlling

Allocation responsibility to each member of the group.

All the members were given equal responsibilities and all performed their role and function as professional.

They manage to reach to the people from small to old with loud and clear voice and variation in presentation with slogans, skits, songs which kept the people grooved till beginning to the end.

Participation of Community

3. Together we can make the effort to keep our environment clean and prevent many diseases (Fig. 3.3). Moreover, have clean surrounding and sanitation; to create awareness, develop healthy attitude. In addition, participate as a group activities geared to solving and minimizing environmental problems.
   - The community has provided with proper data during home visits and interviews.
   - They cooperated with us with active listening and asking relevant questions about the practical problem they were facing.
   - The children were curious and excited to see the carvings and different parts of exhibition thus got the message.

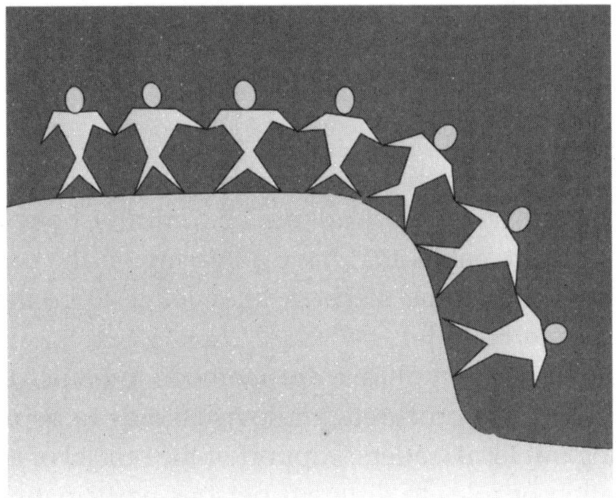

Fig. 3.3: Standing together for health

Since the group used they people language there was better response and interest thus the understood the problem and the message we intanded to pass through.

They asked solution to their problem and we tried to solve their problem with different advices.

Collection of Data/Information Monitoring and Utilization of Data

4. Lack of environmental preservation has ill effect on human kind.
    *   Data was collected through interviews, home visits and clinical nursing process.
    *   Data also as gathered from library books, CHN book, K. Parks 18th edition, internet, newspaper, magazines, and advice from experts, PHC information, etc.

This gave us an insight that if the exhibition is properly organized, attracts large number of people. This gives new ideas to people who stay at remote and do not have access to such information what is good, what is bad, why things otherwise happening, what is the cause, etc. so such mobile small exhibition are effective model of communication, e.g. in fairs and festivals it helps to arouse public conscious.

Public health is important, what misconceptions need to be corrected, what specific attitudes to be developed, what action of the people are desired either a individual or as a village community at large.

All possible information about the problem to be tackled should be collected. To find the community beliefs, local customs, culture habits that have a bearing on the problem.

- Target groups to be reached, knowledge to be imparted, attitudes to be build.
- Facts that need emphasis, apt methods to be used.
- Materials to be procured, audiovisual aids to be used.
- Tracing out local leaders, support of the official of agencies, allocation of roles to different persons participating in the program.

Feasibility of the Project

5. *Source of air pollution* (Fig. 3.4)—Domestic source that is burning of coal, wood, oil; industrial source—factories; automobiles—motor vehicles, railways; others—nuclear explosion.

   Grow vegetables gardens, plant trees, use dust bins, develop healthy habits.

6. Pollution of industrial waste not to put into river or seas (Fig. 3.5). To make different outlet for the industrial waste.
   - Water borne, air borne and soil borne disease can be prevented. It is beneficial to health.
   - The technique and materials used were easily available in local areas.
   - Since people's spoken language was used it was effective.
   - As group studied the real problem that was affecting them and set realistic goals.
   - Therefore, it was feasible to achieve target that was planned.

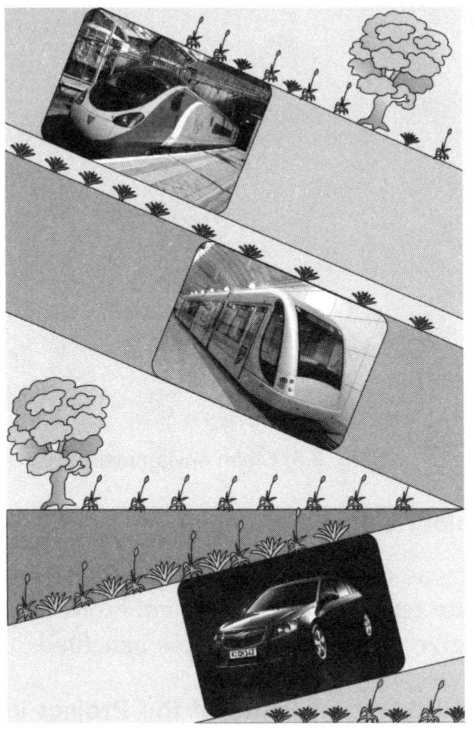

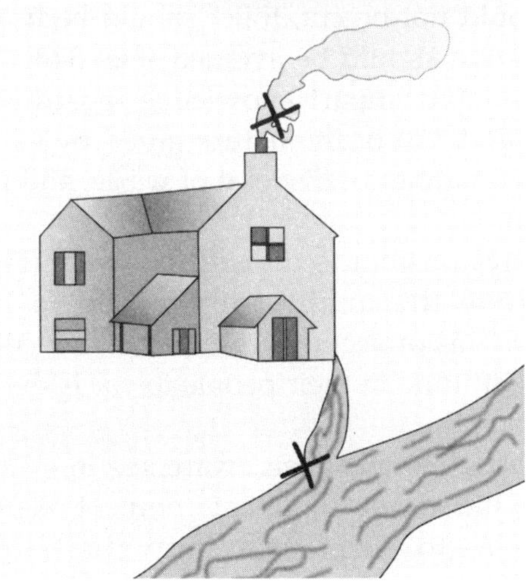

Fig. 3.4: Sources of air pollution

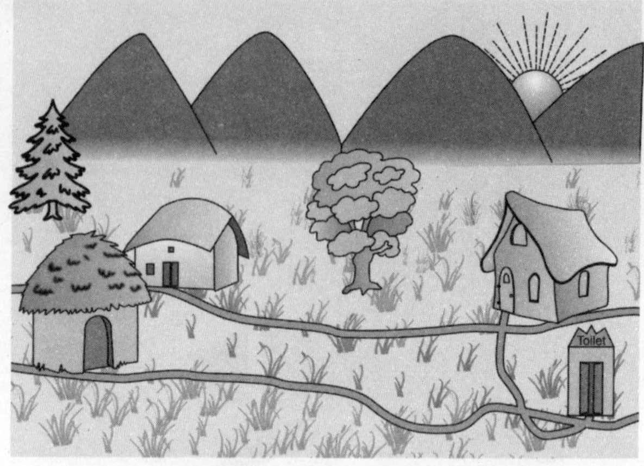

Fig. 3.5: Clean enviornment

Overall Project was Economical

The budget was cost-effective and total cost was minimum with optimum result and achievement. From waste, we made best use to give message and people benefited.

Benefit and Education Value of the Project in Short

7. Trees should not be cut, toilet should be used and open-air defecation should be avoided (Fig. 3.6).
8. To educate and impart knowledge regarding cleanliness (Figs 3.7 and 3.8) of the nature gifted by God and learns the correct manner of disposal of waste, and maintains the sanitation.
9. Use always dustbin to discard the waste (Fig. 3.9).

To improve the quality of life and to live in pure environment. This project makes an effort to inculcate positive and friendly attitude in their people towards the living world around us.

1. *Awareness*—to create an awareness in every individual and in the society about environment related problems.
2. *Attitude*—to help each individual to develop a healthy and positive attitude towards its surrounding he lives.

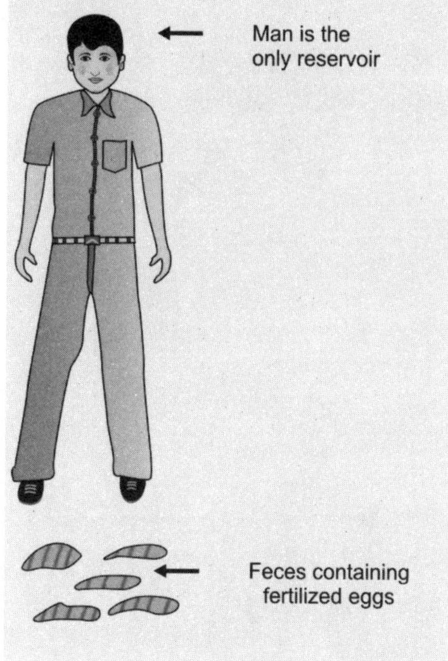

Fig. 3.6: Feces containing fertilized eggs

3. *Knowledge*—to impart knowledge about the essentials values of it and its causes.
4. *Skills*—to inculcate in the students the skills of understanding the need of a healthy environment and develop skills to be sensitive to it to solve the problems.
5. *Participation*—help to provide opportunities to individuals and groups to participate in activities geared to solving or minimizing its problems.

Environmental Problems

10. Human existence cannot be imagined without beauty of natural surrounding, human habits needs to be changed to reduce contamination of soil where, seeding of the soil by ascariasis eggs.

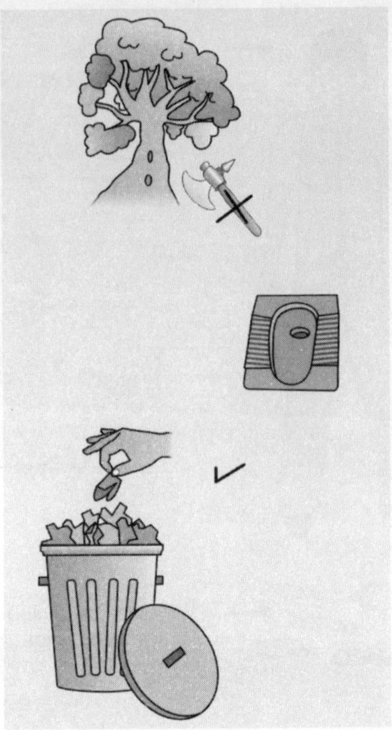

Fig. 3.7: Poster presentation

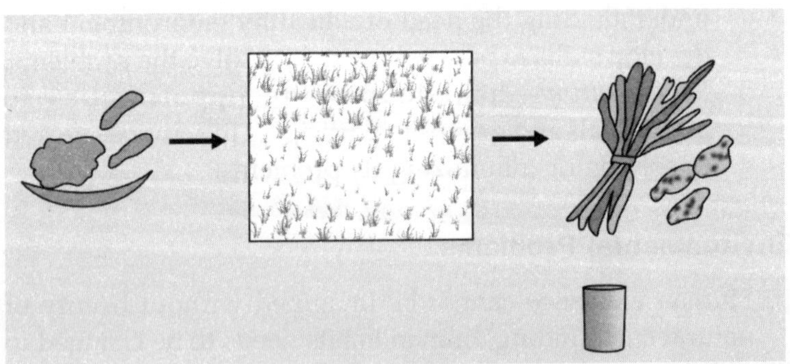

Fig. 3.8: Mode of transmission

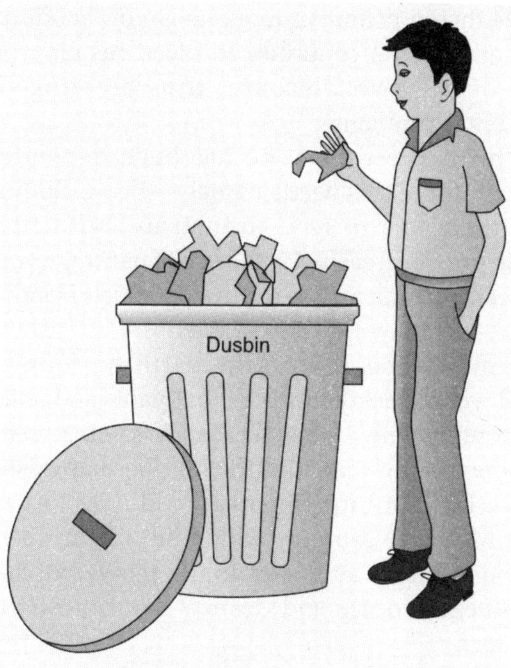

Fig. 3.9: Discarding waste

Takes place by the human habit of unsanitary disposal of human excreta.

11. How can a threat to the atmosphere be reduced? To realize the danger and take a step to reduce the risk factor. Human excreta are a source of infection. About 98% of the people in rural areas use open fields for defecation. These practices are harmful for health.

To bring awareness that feces is infectious, pollutes water and soil, and promotes fly breading, worm infestation, etc. when man first appeared on our planet earth, the entire globe was with lots of animals and plants—all living in complete harmony with the natural and ever beautiful environment. Man being a superior being started challenging the laws of nature. He multiplied in number at the expense of the plants and animal's that formed his environment.

He was then a primitive man, he is now modern and well educated and yet he continues to bleed his environment for the sake of his own pleasure, thus creating unwanted environmental problem.

From his earliest days, he has been dependent on his environment for all his needs namely—Food, clothing, shelter and raw materials to feed industries. With time human population grew increasingly, the use of natural resources went beyond a certain limit and harmful side effects began to become evident.

When man appeared on the earth he found him in a wonderful world thickly inhabited by plants and animals living in total harmony with each other. Sad to say that man was then more superior being than all forms of life that existed then.

He was far more intelligent as well. He lost no time to challenge Mother Nature of which he was an offspring. He considered himself as a dominant master of nature and ruthlessly began to use and destroy nature resources for his own comfort.

Thus begun the process of pollution of our own biosphere. Intelligent as man still is, it is time that he realizes that excessive pollution will eventually suffocate life on earth and so it is about time that serious steps are taken to undo the harm done through and to stop further damage to the mother earth.

How can threats to the atmosphere are reduced.

Having realized the danger we have put our nature, we must now take step to reduce the risk factor and do things that will help regain as much as of its previous glory as possible.

Steps to be Taken

12. Soil pollution affects human by worm infestation. Through open air defecation (Fig. 3.10) and walking barefooted. Life cycle of worm infestation and transmission through various mode of unhygienic and lack of personal hygienic practice (Fig. 3.11).

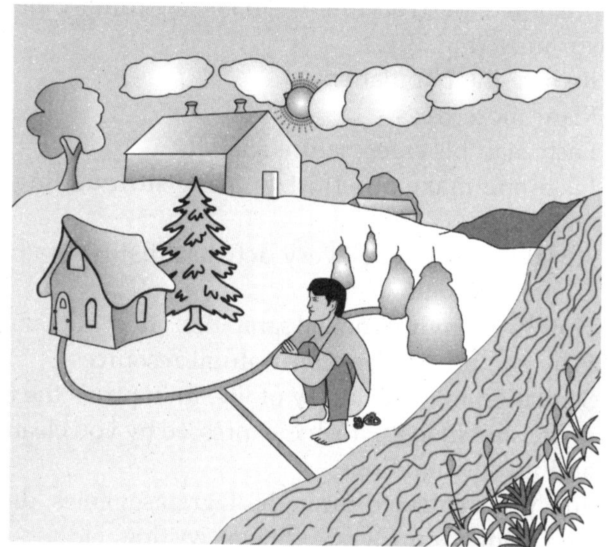

Fig. 3.10: Open air defecation

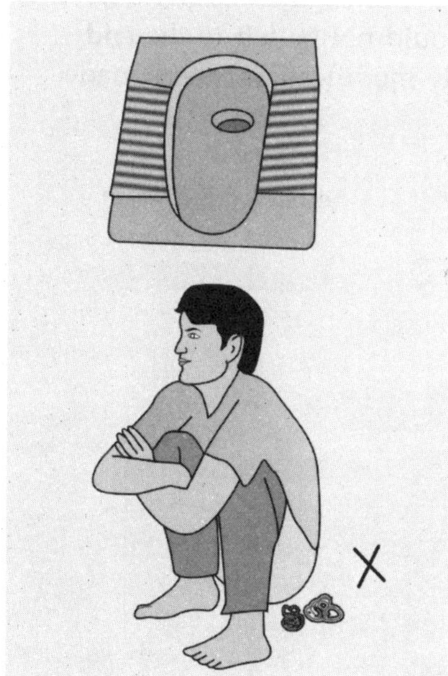

Fig. 3.11: Using toilets instead of open defecation

Importance of treatment—mass treatment periodic deworming (Fig. 3.12).

- Reduce the population.
- Plant more trees.
- Each man becomes nature friendly.
- Each one make an effort to make surrounding green and clean.
- All avoid any and every act that disturbes environmental sanitation.
- How does environmental sanitation affect human being?
- Why should we conserve natural resources?
- Sanitation to make a way of life, to improve the quality of life, and living, which is expressed by you clean home and its surroundings.

All this was explained through diagrams, games, dramas/skit, made things from waste, slogan writing, etc.

If exhibition is prepared and organized according to aims and objectives, it can attract large number of people. Evaluation should not be left to the end

Successfully modification can be made.

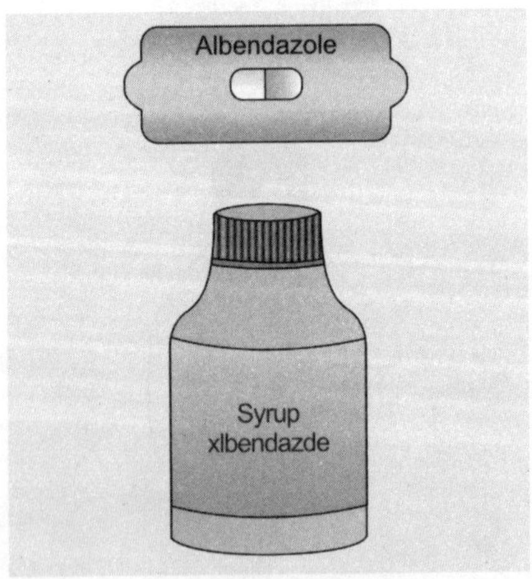

Fig. 3.12: Medicines

Group Presentation

Definition as above

13. Creating awareness and motivating people for environmental sanitation and its good results in health and happiness.

    Spread this message to rural fields, schools, etc (Fig. 3.13).

    Spread the message that every man on earth becomes nature friendly. Each human being makes his surrounding green. All avoid every act that pollutes air and environment and conserve natural resources.

Importance of Environmental Health

In modern concept, environment includes not only the water, air and soil that form our environment but also the social, economic condition under which we live.

Much of ill health in India is due to poor environmental sanitation, that is unsafe water, polluted soil, unhygienic disposal of human excreta and refuse, poor housing, insects and rodents.

Therefore, it is crucial to prevent diseases and promote health as large number of people in India lives in rural areas we stressed sanitation factors that are harmful to health.

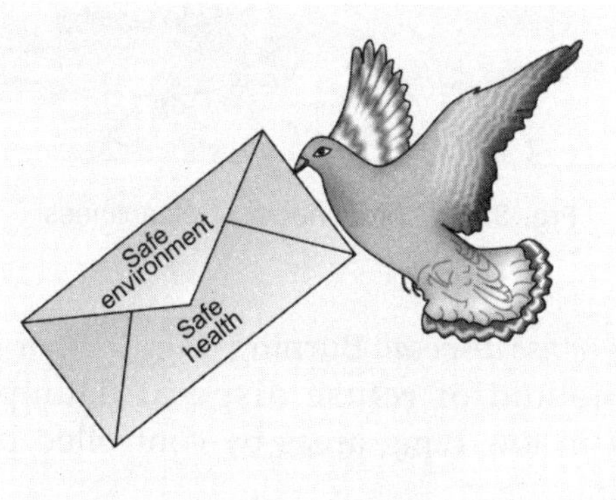

Fig. 3.13: Spread message

Components

Physical—water, soil, housing, radiation.

14. Clean hands, clean water, clean air, are signs of good sanitation, therefore, hand washing before and after defecation, cutting nails short and drinking boiled water will enhance sanitary habits (Fig. 3.14).

    Biological—plants and animals life including bacteria, virus, insects, rodents.

    Social—Customs, culture, habits, income, occupation, religion, etc.

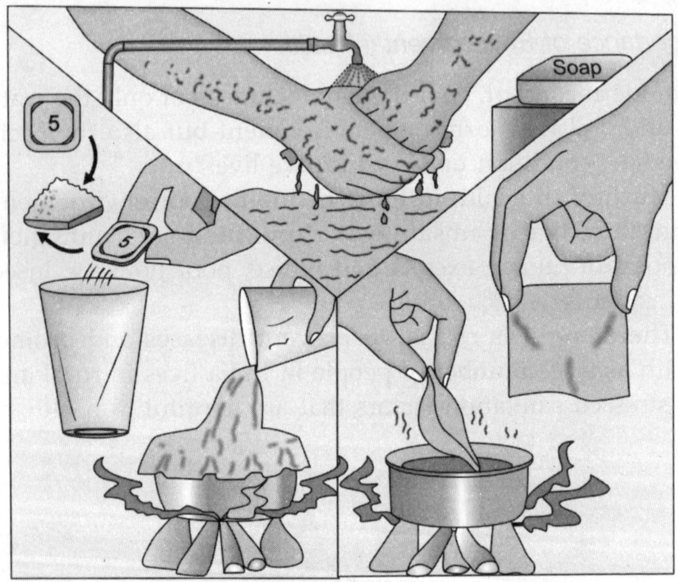

Fig. 3.14: Components of cleanliness

15. *Method of refuse disposal*: Burning (Fig. 3.15) or incineration is best method of refuse disposal. Dump refuse by dumping in low-lying areas by controlled pipping and composting.

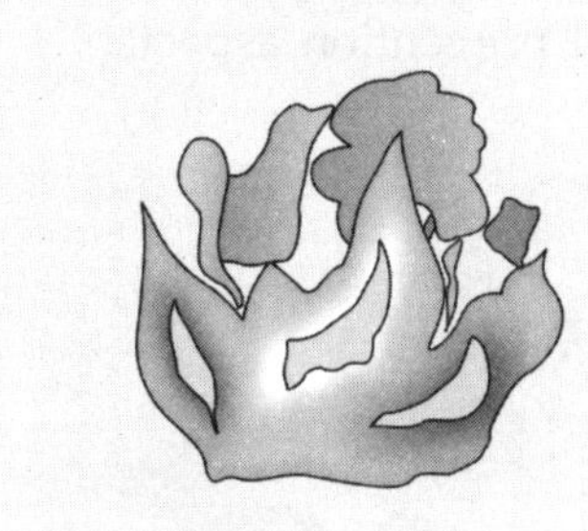

Fig. 3.15: Burning of waste

16. What is drop of water? Every drop of water (Fig. 3.16) is precious.
Where there is water there life blooms and blossoms forth.
Every drop of water makes the ocean.
Value—preserving water.

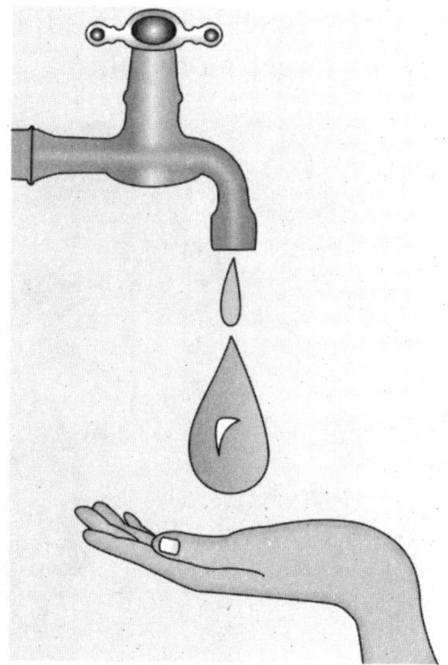

Fig. 3.16: Drop of water

17. Do not cut the trees (Fig. 3.17)
    Components and prevention aspects.

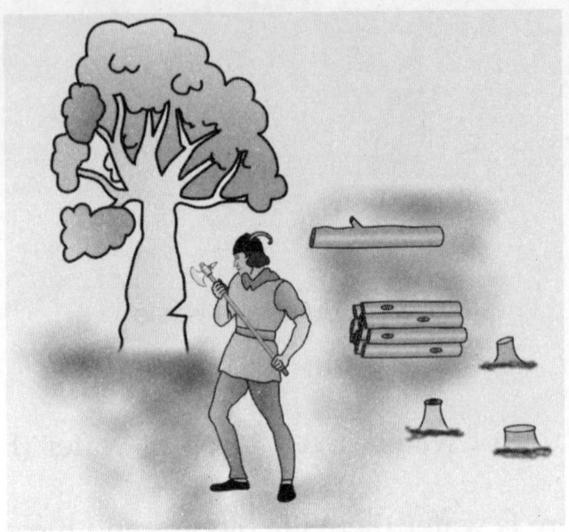

Fig. 3.17: Cutting trees

18. Clean surrounding (Fig. 3.18) which enhances health. Moreover, it improves well-being. In addition; a tree gives beauty, shed, helps to get more rain.

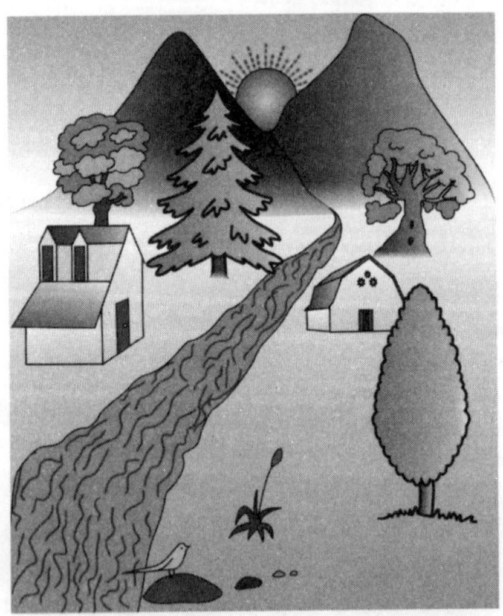

Fig. 3.18: Clean surrounding

19. *Signs and symptoms of unclean environmental sanitation:*
    In addition, its ill effect on human being, effects of noise pollution such as deafness, interference with speech, inability to concentrate, loss of speech, disturbances in sleep, accidents in industries, physiological changes like high blood pressure, etc.

    More than 100 substances pollute air like carbon dioxide, carbon monoxide, and sulphur dioxide, cancer producing substances, dust and smoke.

    Health effects (Figs 3.19 and 3.20) are immediate and delayed, e.g. acute bronchitis, suffocation, lung cancer, etc.

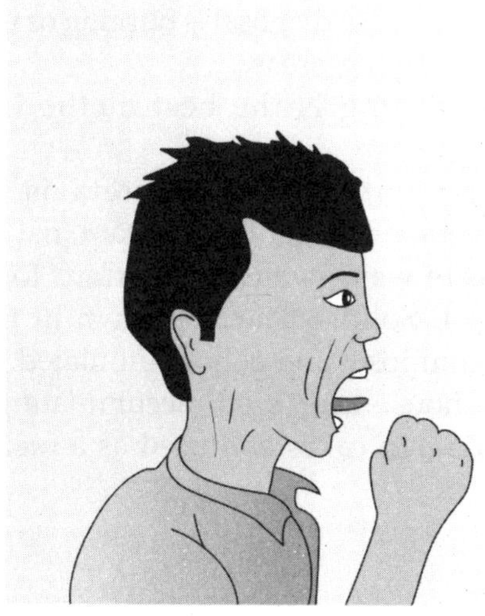

Fig. 3.19: Coughing

20. Effect of environmental pollution on health.
    Water—It is the main source through which all the water-borne diseases are spread. It can be prevented by boiling water and filled in domestic filter.

    Rural man thinks that latrines are meant for city dwellers, where there are no fields for defecation. He is ignorant that feces are infecting water and soil and promoting fly and diseases.

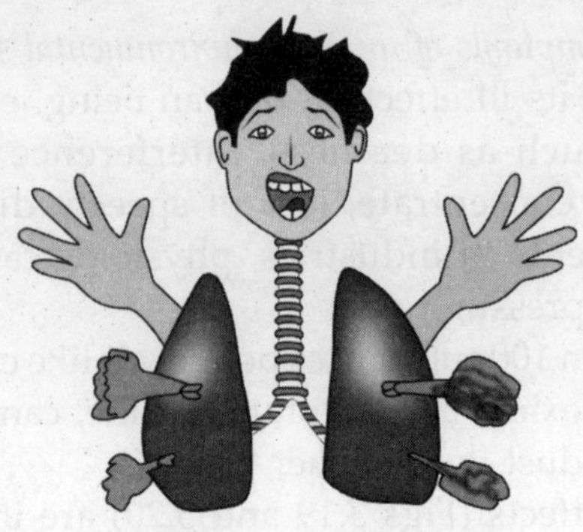

Fig. 3.20: Lung disease

The best method of refuse disposal is burning or incineration. Dumping it in low-lying areas.

Controlled pipping is the best method for refuse disposal.

Refuse along with human excreta is known as composting. The average villager is not aware that mosquitoes breed in collections of waste-water. He permits to flow waste often into the street. Solid waste is thrown in front of the houses where it decomposes and gets accumulated. The animal dung too near the house keep's on accumulating. It can be sun dried and made into cakes and used as a fuel which is a good habit.

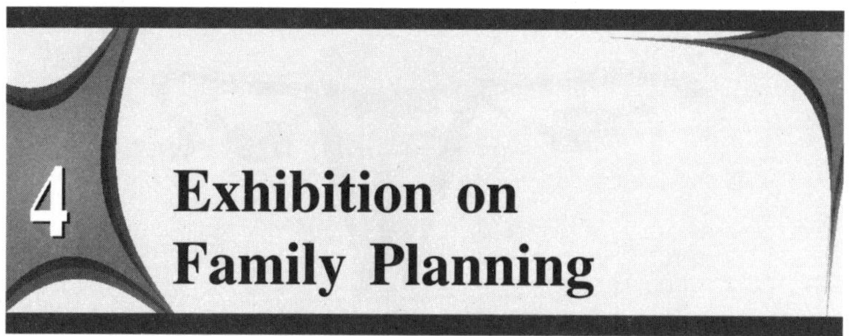

Exhibition on Family Planning

MODERN METHODS OF FAMILY PLANNING

It is defined as the way of thinking and living that is adopted voluntarily upon the basis of knowledge attitudes and responsible decisions by the individual and couples, in order to promote the health and welfare of family; groups and thus contribute effectively to the social development of the country.

Method Condom/Nirodh (Fig. 4.1)

The condom is a thin rubber sheath used by men during sex. It is a cover made of rubber, designed to be placed on the penis just before sexual intercourse. They are supplied free of cost in government health centers. Easily available through commercial outlets, easy to use, protects from unwanted pregnancy, protects against STDs and AIDS and no side effects. The condom must be put on after full erection. The condom prevents the deposition of semen in the vagina. Condom should not be reused.

Sterilization Operation-Women (Fig. 4.2)

It is permanent, once performed woman no longer has children. It is used as permanent contraceptives measure when a couple has already had a large number of children. It requires an abdominal operation. Hospitalization is required for 5 to 7 days.

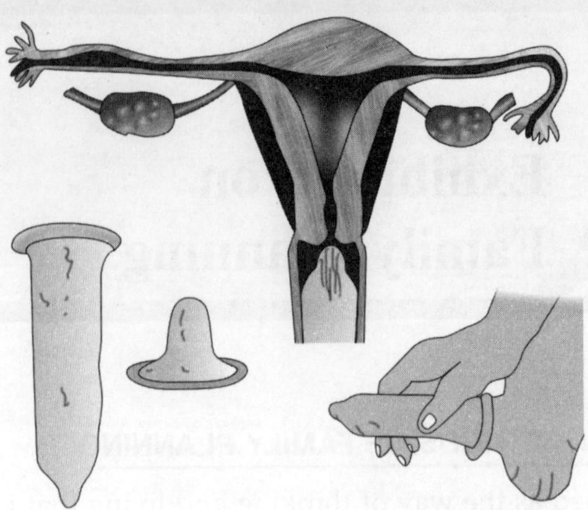

Fig. 4.1: Method Condom/nirodh

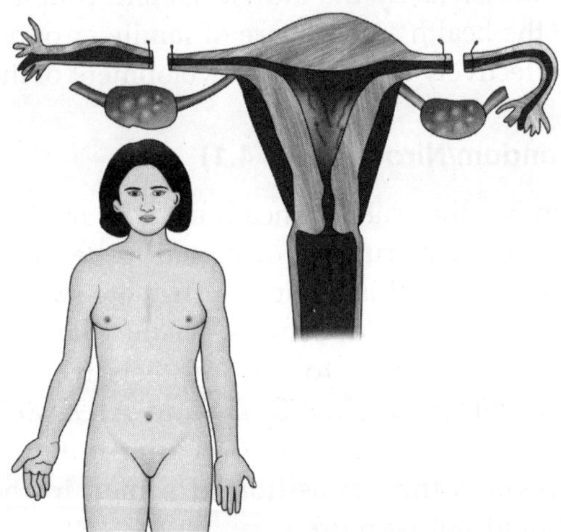

Fig. 4.2: Sterilization operation

Vaginal Diaphragm

It is a soft rubber dome with a coiled spring ring. It is inserted into the vagina prior to intercourse where, it covers the cervix completely and prevents the spermatozoa from entering the uterus. It must remain in place for at least 6 hours after

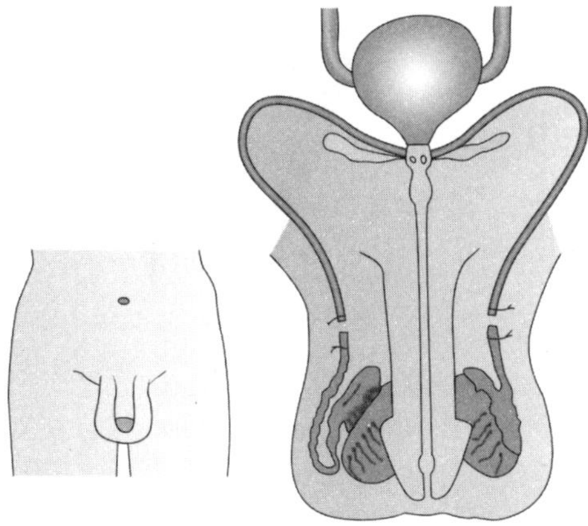

Fig. 4.3: In men (vasectomy)

intercourse. For better effectiveness, a contraceptive jelly, cream should be also used.

Foam Tablets, Creams and Jellies

A measured quality and quantity of cream or jelly is introduced into the vagina by a special applicator just before sexual intercourse. At body temperature, they melt and spread in the vagina and provide a thin film of a chemical barrier (Fig. 4.4).

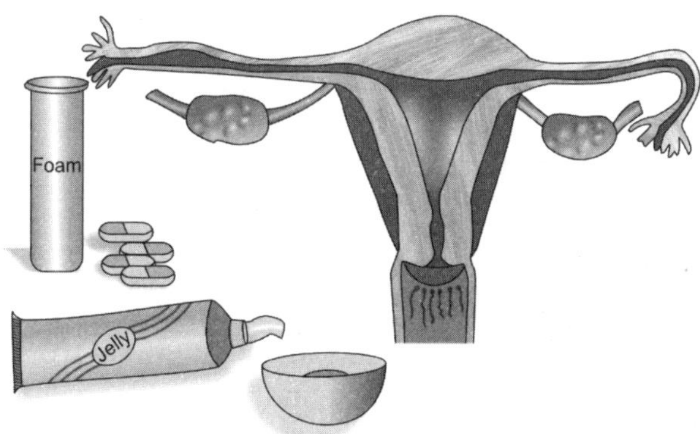

Fig. 4.4: Foam, creams and jellies

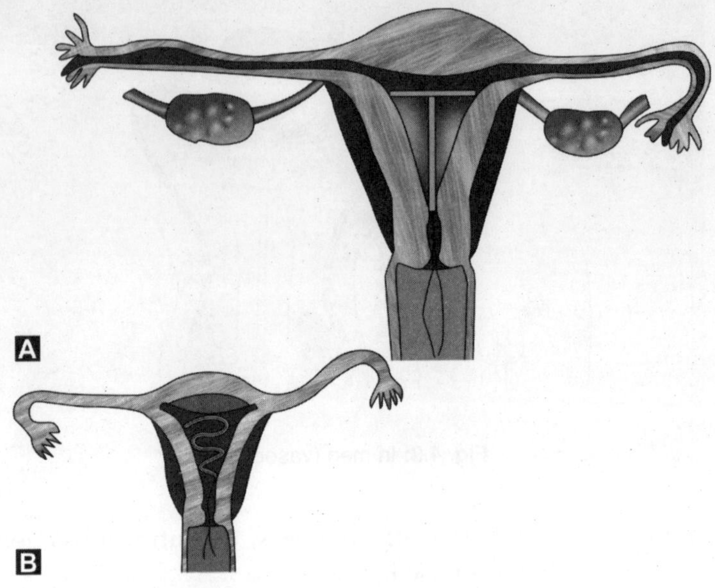

Figs 4.5A and B: A Copper T, B-Lippes loop

Intrauterine Devices/IUD

Copper T- is made of plastic material and copper wire is wrapped around the stem of the device. Since copper can dissolve slowly, the copper T may be replaced every 3 to 5 years. It is not interfering with normal sex life of the wearer. It is easy to insert, less pain and bleeding and greater effective results (Fig. 4.5A).

Lippes loop is double S-shaped plastic device made of polyethylene. It has attached threads or tails made of nylon. The best time for IUD insertion is between 3 to 7 days of menstruation cycle (Fig 4.5B).

Hormonal Contraceptives (Figs 4.6A and B)

Oral pills contain small amounts of an estrogen and progesterone. They are effective and reversible method. They prevent pregnancy by inhibiting ovulation.

Types of pills like Mala-N and Mala-D. Mode of intake is a packet of oral pills contains 28 pills, of which 21 are

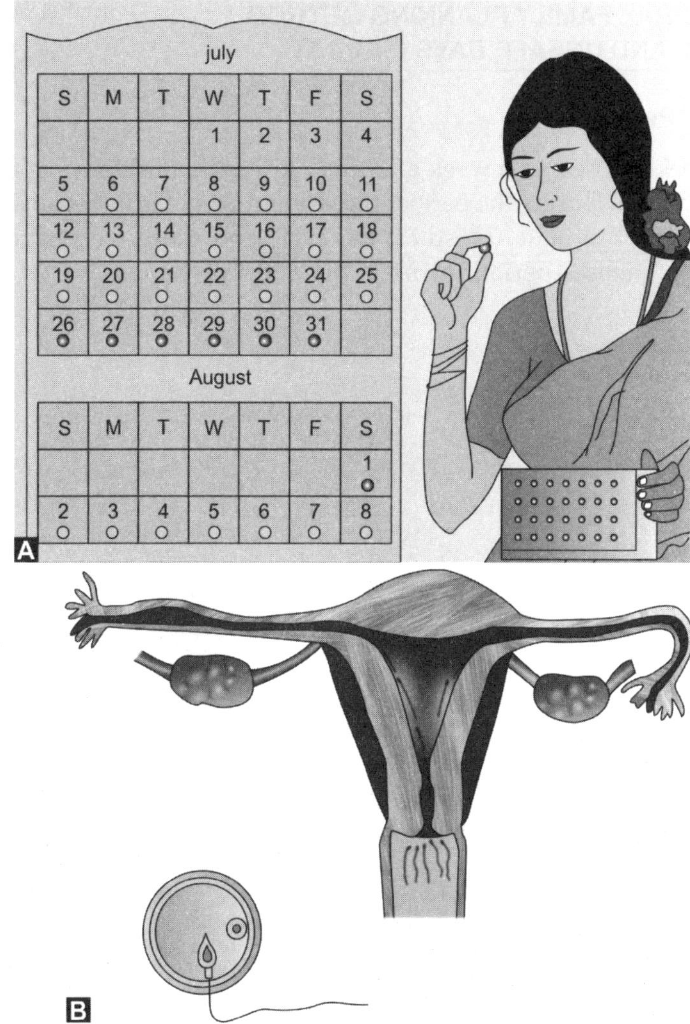

Figs 4.6A and B: Hormonal contraceptives

contraceptive and 7 are iron tablets. The first course of the pill should be started on the 5th day of menstruation as day one. Daily one tablet should be taken as indicated on packet in arrow. As packet is finished, next day new packets should be started. The pill should be taken daily at fixed time in mainly at night.

NATURAL FAMILY PLANNING METHOD
SAFE AND UNSAFE DAYS (FIG. 4.7)

Safe Period

A week before and a week after the menses is considered as a safe period. During the period, the woman is not fertile because she cannot ovulate. To study the cycle and those who have regular menses period learns fertile and safe period.

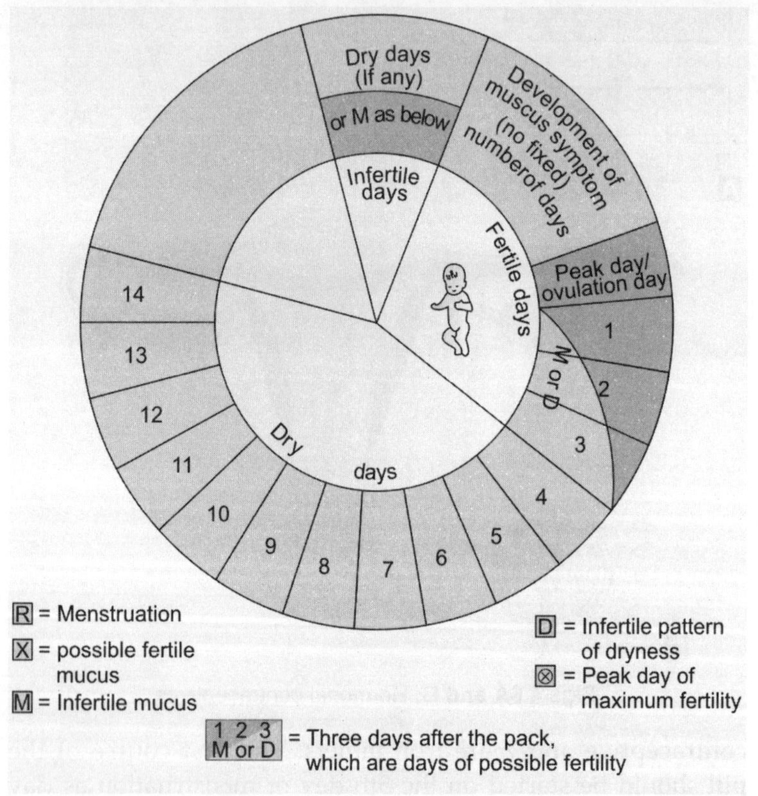

Fig. 4.7: Natural family planning method. safe and unsafe days

Natural Family Planning And Safe and Unsafe Days of Fertility (Figs 4.8A to C)

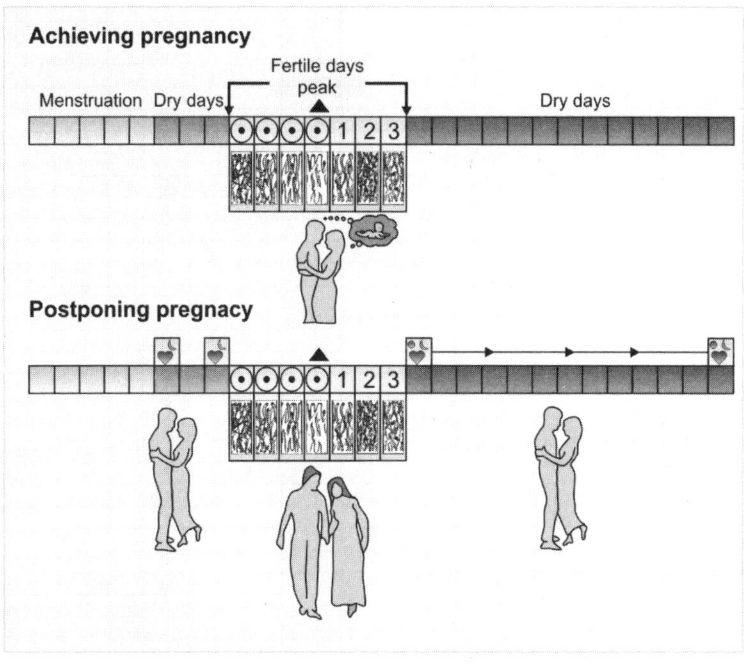

Fig. 4.8A: Natural family planning and safe and unsafe days of fertility

Billings Ovulation Method Chart

NAME:

Cycle day	1	2	3	4	5	6	7	8	9	10	11	12	13	14	15	16	17	18	19	20	21	22	23	24	25	26	27	28	29	30	31	32	33	34	35
Date																																			
Symbol																																			
Remarks: Describe feeling and appearance of mucus.																																			
Cycle day																																			
Date																																			
Symbol																																			
Remarks:																																			
Cycle day																																			
Date																																			
Symbol																																			
Remarks:																																			
Cycle day																																			
Date																																			
Symbol																																			
Remarks:																																			

Symbol:
R or Red Menstruation,
D or green-dry days
X or no colour days when mucus is stretchy, slippery changing, wet and clear like raw egg white
(X)-peak dya
1,2,3-post peak days
D-Dry days

Possible remarks
Wet, slippery, stretchy, stringy flaky, pasty, cloudy, dry, clear, pain,

Note:
Day 1 is the first day of menstruation. Write the MONTH involved after the word DATE then fill in the dates.

Fig. 4.8B: Ovulation chart and changes in body temperature

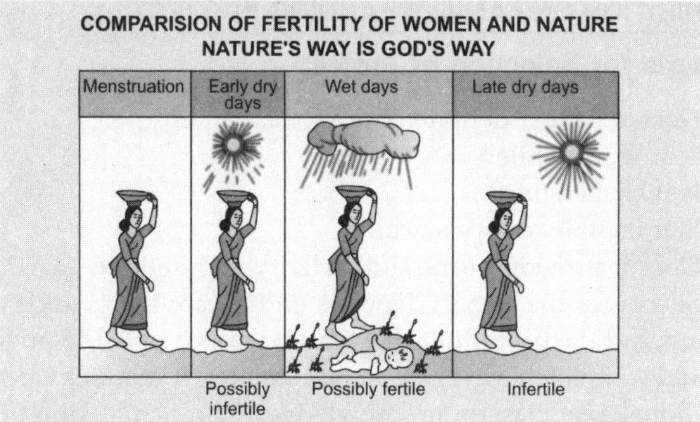

Fig. 4.8C: Natural way of family planning

Mucus Method Study and Self-Examination

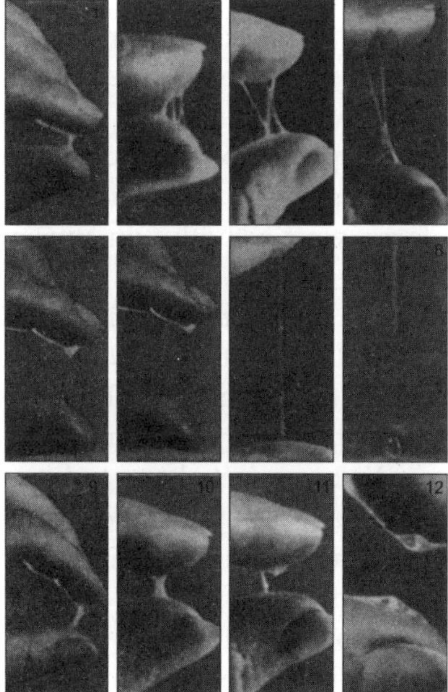

Fig. 4.9: Key to fertility control:the mucus

EXHIBITION ON FAMILY PLANNING PROJECT

Criteria for Selection of Project

- Does it have a definite educational value?
- Is it worthwhile?
- Is it challenging?
- Is it feasible and practical?
- Does it provide purposeful activity and definite goals?

Success of the project depends on the care with which the details and the procedures have been worked out. The project should completely cover the subject matter. It requires careful planning. Use classroom knowledge to an actual situation. Topic selected should have educational value and must be adapted to the needs of the situation.

Your planning determines the future course of action. You have to keep in mind what is to be done, how is to be done, when is to be done, where is to be done.

Your group plan will precede other functions. Your success of group project depends on your effective planning. Planning will help you to coordinate, control, and lead to completeness of action. It should be precise and measurable. Clarity in the direction of activities.

Chalk out the sequence of steps and avoid overlapping and duplication. Adapt to the situation, make use of available resources and focus your activities on aims and objectives of the project.

Form also general statement of policies which will provide guide, it should be directed to your objectives and you will be able to maintain stability and flexibility.

The steps to be taken, the resources to be used, your concrete scheme. Your projects have to be materialized into action. For that you need group members, time, target, money, which is not an abstract through in mind but measurable, e.g. a blue print of your plan.

Match limited resources with need, problems and situation, eliminate waste resources; it is a teamwork.

Project is Individual and Group

The class as a unit, e.g. making a model—Learning project like learning to make a fracture bed, learn to operate monitor in ICCU.

Intellectual Project

A nursing student who is caring of a patient with low hemoglobin finds that her patient seems to be mentally confused. The patient is given blood plasma and the mental confusion disappears immediately, e.g. find out the causes of hypoglycemia and explain the importance of timing of meals.

- Physical and maternal project, e.g. safe motherhood model/
- Project can be demonstrated, exhibited, conducted mini health fair seminar, group discussion, puppet show, role-play, CD-video presentation.
- Can be conducted ANC, PNC, OPD, CLINIC, industries, old age home, urban schools, rural anganwadies and mahilamandals
- Only it should be self-motivated, goal-directed and teachers approval.
- To find out the reason for the sudden change may become an intellectual project for a student.
- The project is a valuable method of teaching.

In Group Project

All members should have a common understanding of the goals towards which they are working.

Goals Set up by Group

- Group members have to learn to become maximally effective in the performance of skills relevant to their goals.
- All should participate in all the aspects of group functioning.
- Evaluation will help to learn how effectively they are working towards goal.
- It demand careful placing and considerable social skill.

- It should be on burning problem.
- It should be on national problem.
- It should be based on educational needs of students.
- Related to health aspect.
- Feasible and practical.
- Social background of beneficiary.

GROUP PROJECT MODEL-I

Exhibition on Family Planning

"DELAY THE FIRST, POSTPONE THE SECOND AND PREVENT THE THIRD" (Figs 4.10A to D)

Members of the group
1.
2.
3.
4.
Title of the project—Family planning.

Introduction

This is a project on "family planning" which deals with the different types of methods which are used for family planning

We have taken this topic to educate the people about the methods that are used for family planning and make the group of people understand about the advantages of the recent methods of family planning.

Family planning clarifies that the ultimate goal is social development of the country and above all to create a happy family.

The WHO has given the following definition about family planning as "the way of thinking and living that is adopted voluntarily upon the bases of knowledge attitudes and responsible decisions by the individual and couples, in order to promote the health and welfare of family, groups and thus contribute effectively to the social development of the country". Form of project— exhibition—Standing together for health.

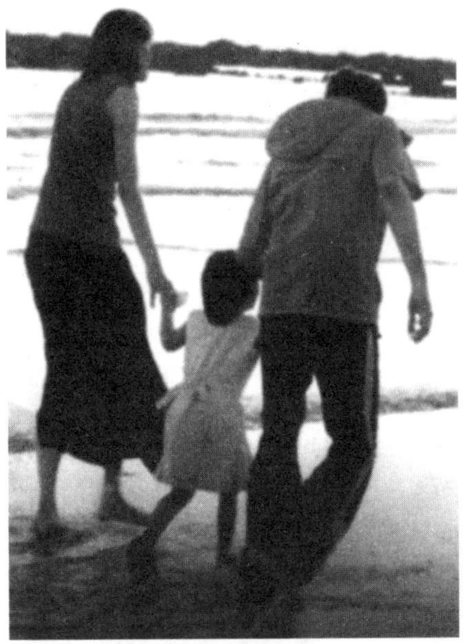

Fig. 4.10A: Happy family

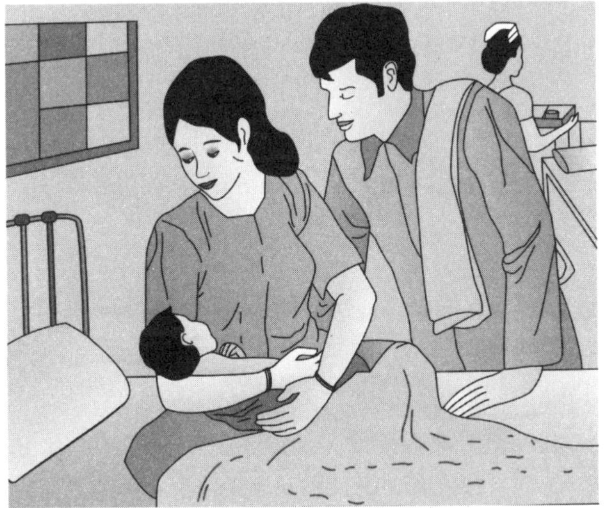

Fig. 4.10B: Hum do-humara ek the symbol of family

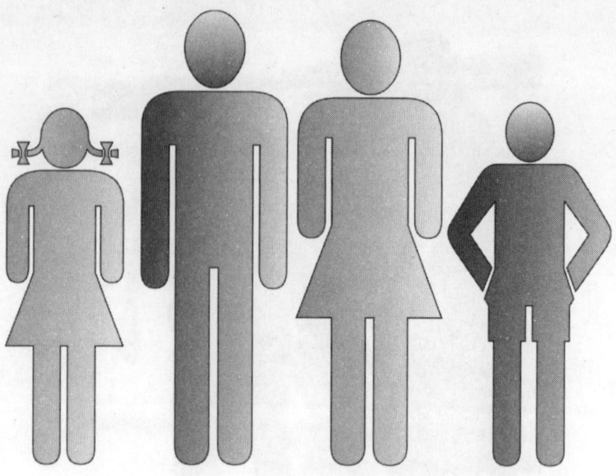

Fig. 4.10C: Delay the first, postpone the second and prevent the third

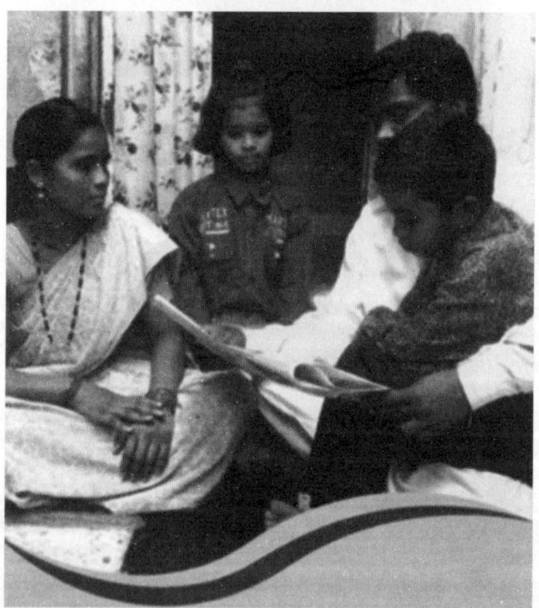

Fig. 4.10D: Hum do humare do

Type of Project

Light, flexible, portable, carriable and easy to shift and assemble from the institution to the field area.

Name of the institution

Year of student:

Name of the group

1.

2.

3.

4.

5.

Date of completion of project:

Name of the teacher:

Need for the project:

- For promoting health and family welfare in the country through education, training.
- To create awareness.
- To increase the motivation and cooperation of people and to control the increasing population.
- Due to population explosion, few job opportunities.
- Inadequate school facilities.
- A high percentage of illiteracy.
- Lack of substandard housing.
- Over crowding.
- Political dissatisfaction.
- High IMR and MMR.
- Lower expectation of life.
- Low level of nutrition.
- Better health facilities.
- Delay marriage.
- Premarital sex education.
- Environmental hazards, pollution of water, food and soil.
- Poor quality of health services.
- Living under poverty line leads to sickness and sickness into poverty and goes on vicious circle of its numberless consequences.

- Keeping this above entire needs in mind, we have selected this project, to boost the target achievements.

Planning of the Project

This project was planned out to educate and impart knowledge regarding family planning. The group members planned to play a skit and slogans showing problems and needs of small family and a big family. It aims to give quality of life and promote small family two-child norm using FP methods and clinical services. Plan to stabilize population to establish small family size.

We decided to explain the temporary methods of family planning with demonstration and permanent methods with charts and flash cards and the different models we had prepared. We also decided to explain the advantages and disadvantages of each method. For creating awareness, we planned so sing one "jagruti song" and a theme song prepared by the groups creativity.

We also decided that each group member would be involved and give their best for making the project reach out to people in community and making the project successful.

Preplan

1. Background information of the area.
2. Rural field posting of the students— Parol is a small village located in Thane district. The houses mostly are built "kachcha" very few homes have electricity and sanitary latrines available. The people have lack of knowledge about "family planning" as illiteracy is more in this area. There is increase in number of children in the family and so on, etc.
3. Survey, if any—according to the data collected from the family survey, we came to know that there is increase in number of children in the family. Malnutrition, anemia, early marriage, illiteracy and dropouts among school going children was present.

There are many other health problems prevalent. There is poor maintenance of personal hygiene and poor environmental sanitation.

We also came to know that the people in this area are mostly using temporary methods but they are unaware about the permanent sterilization methods. Untrained personnel's do mostly deliveries at home, registration of birth, marriage were delayed.

Therefore, we fixed the priority of this project in order that the family welfare becomes a people centered program.

Goals

1. To promote the adoption of small family size norm; on the basis of voluntary acceptance" hum do humare do".
2. To promote the use of spacing methods/spacing children at least three years apart (fertility period 15 to 45).
3. To ensure adequate supply of contraceptives to all eligible couples within each reach.
4. To arrange for clinical and surgical services so as to archive the set targets.
5. Reduce IMR and MMR.
6. Delay marriage, preferably after 20 years.
7. Achieve 80% institutional deliveries by 100% trained Dai.
8. Improve the life expectancy of female.
9. Increase literacy rate.
10. Control and prevent unwanted births because health of the family also depends on the size of the family.

Development of family planning in India—explain the concept of how family planning concept was developed.
1. 1877 Dr Annie who raised the issue and introduced family planning service before the public.
2. 1925 professor, Larvee Mumbai started propaganda on birth control.
3. 1930 Mysore Government started the birth control clinic.
4. 1935 Indian Congress favored the family planning program.
5. 1951 comprehensive program to check rapid population growth.

6. 1953, 147 family planning clinics set up.
7. 1969 Rs. 315 million allocated to family planning.

Objectives

Family planning refers to practices that help individuals and couples to attain certain objectives:
1. To avoid unwanted births.
2. To bring about wanted births.
3. To regulate the intervals between pregnancies.
4. To control the time at which births occur in relation to the ages of the parent.
5. To determine the number of children in the family.

Assessment of Resources

1. The resources used were very effective.
2. Chart papers were used to make posters.
3. The thermocol used were cheap and of good quality.
4. Posters were also used.
5. Some other resources like condom, Mala-N, Mala-D, were used. These were brought as a sample to show the people in the community.
6. To collect the data and matter for family planning we made use of many books, magazines and newspapers, etc. to get more information about it.
7. Pins were used to give support to the thermacol, and clay was used for models.
8. Cardboards were used to show some of the temporary methods.
9. Fevicol was used for sticking.
10. Sketch pens and watercolors were used.

Fixing of Priority

Today in India, population explosion has been increasing and so efforts should be made by us to control the population growth. So, family planning should be adopted in every Indian family to control the population growth. In order to bring awareness about family planning and to motivate the people for adopting family planning methods' we wanted people to know the various contraceptive methods available; we choose "family panning" as our main topic for the group project.

Expected Outcome of the Project

According to the last census taken, India ranks second in the world; in terms of population growth. Day by day India's population is increasing. Population explosion is the boosting major problem of our country because of which there is scarcity of resources leading to hazards like increase in poverty, illiteracy, unemployment, crimes and health problems affecting the whole country.

To promote good health facilities to the people and to reduce the hazards of increasing population the Government of India is trying to reach the message of small family norm "Hum Do Humare Do", or "Hum Do Humara Ek."

As India is known "The land of villages", villages play a vital role in every aspect of our country.

Therefore, Government of India is trying to make efforts for population control and family planning especially in villages. There is lack of knowledge, illiteracy and lack of awareness in the people living in villages, Govt is trying to provide information about family planning to the last village, to the last family, to the last person.

As the proverb says, "Prevention is better than cure." In order to prevent the occurrence of many diseases, we should control the population growth.

Each of our group members made best efforts to provide information and awareness to motivate the people for population control by making use of family planning methods. and the end pamphlet and literature on family planning was distributed.

Implementation

Resource Available

The resource that was available is as follows:
Charts, flashcards, posters, thermocol, cardboards, mount boards, clay, educational literature, samples available for temporary methods of contraception like condom, Copper-T, Mala-N, Mala-D, pins, Fevicol, gum, sketch pens, water colors, cotton swabs, pen, pencil, etc.

Manpower Required

For example— There were seven members in our group.
- Introduction about the explanation and explained about 'Mala - N' and Slogans.
- Explained about condoms and explained how to control spread of AIDS, objectives and goals of family planning.
- Explained about Diaphragm.
- Explained Copper-T, Lippes loop, Tubectomy using thermocol carving.
- Explained about Rhythm Method.
- Explained about insertion of Copper - T using thermocol carving.
- Explained about vasectomy (Fig. 4.3).

Equipment Required

The equipment used were charts, flashcards, posters, thermocol, cardboards, mount boards, pins, Fevicol, gum, sketch pens, water colors, cotton swabs, pen, pencil; samples which were available for temporary methods of contraception like condom, Copper-T, Mala - N, Mala - D, etc.

Appropriate Technology

Lectures and Discussion
The technology used were:

- First we explained the introduction about "Family Planning".
- Then we performed a role play showing a small family and a big family.
- Then we explained the various family planning methods through demonstration using.
  Thermocol carving, flashcards and charts.

Organization

1. Work Place: Rural area—Parol
2. Schedule of Stages: Evening 5 pm to 7-30 pm.

Start to Finish—used Properly

- Introduction about family planning.
- Definition.
- Goals and objectives.
- Types of Family Planning Methods.
- Types of temporary methods of contraception for males and females.
- Advantages and disadvantages of both temporary and permanent methods of contraception
- Role play.
- Jagruti song, slogans.

Controlling

Allocated Responsibility to Each Members of Group

There were seven members in our group; each group member was allocated different works. The responsibilities were:

- Introduce about family planning and to explain about 'Mala - N'.
- Explaining about condoms and objectives and goals of family planning.
- Explaining diaphragm.
- Explaining Copper - T, Lippes loop, Tubectomy.
- Explaining about Rhythm Method.

- Explaining insertion of Copper - T using thermocol carving and conclusion.
- Explaining vasectomy.

Collection of Data

Family surveys, textbooks, newspapers, magazines, internet and other references from library, and pamphlet and literature from PHC.

Information Monitoring and Utilization of Data

According to family survey, we collected information and data from various books and other available like condom, Mala-N, Copper-T, etc. We decided to make use of easy language so that people can easily understand.

Appropriate Technology

- Lectures and discussion.
- First we explained what Family Planning is?
- We then performed a Role Play.
- We explained the various family planning methods through demonstration using. Thermocol carving and charts.

Participation of Community

- The group of people participated actively.
- Men and women of all ages were gathered for the exhibition.
- School going children were gathered in a huge numbers. They all were excited to see all the charts, flashcards, thermocol carving, and they enjoyed the role play that we performed in front of the people.
- Besides the role play they also enjoyed the Jagruti Song.
- The group of people was quietly listening to what all our three groups were explaining.

Overall Project was Economical: Low cost, lot of waste from best method was used

Yes, our project was economical.

Thermocol	:	Rs. 33
Mount board	:	Rs. 10
Fevicol	:	Rs. 13
Sketch pens	:	Rs. 15
Chart papers	:	Rs. 21
Cello sticking	:	Rs. 10
Balloons	:	Rs. 12
Stickers	:	Rs. 10
Plastic cover	:	Rs. 12
Total	:	Rs. 136

Benefit to Community

The people in the community lacked knowledge regarding 'Family Planning'. Therefore, we decided to teach people 'Family Planning' in the form of project and in the exhibition.

The people were benefited as project provided them with the following:
- Information about family planning.
- Temporary methods of family planning in men and women
- Permanent methods of family planning in men and women
- Hazards of population growth we made aware to the people
- Advantages and disadvantages of increase population growth.

Education Value of the Project

- The community people understood the various family planning methods and the important of adopting family planning in order to control the population growth.

- Because of the project work and exhibition, we ourselves improved our knowledge regarding various Health Education to the villages "for serving people is serving God.

Innovative Approach

- Advised people not to practice, "Early Marriage" and "Child Marriages."
- Encouraged people to maintain good health through 'Good Nutrition'.
- Motivated people to adopt 'Family Planning.'
- Various information regarding all of the methods of contraception were provided to people.
- Encouraged people to adopt the 'Small Family Norm', e.g. 'Hum Do, Humare Do.'

Group Presentation of Project

Definition

The WHO has defined "Family Planning" as "The way of thinking and living that is adopted voluntarily upon the basis of knowledge attitudes and responsible decisions by the individual and couples, in order to promote the health and welfare of family, groups and thus contribute effectively to the social development of the county.

Contraceptive

Contraceptive means preventing:
a. The union of sperm and ovum
b. Suppressing ovulation
c. Interfering with implantation of the fertilized ovum in the uterus.

Classification of Contraceptive Methods

a. For Men: (Temporary Methods):
   1. Condom
   2. Withdrawal.

b. For Women:
1. Intrauterine Devices
   - Lippes loop
   -. Copper - T.
2. Hormonal Contraceptives
   - Oral
   - Injectable
   - Subdermal.
3. Diaphragms
4. Foam tablets, jelly and cream
5. Rhythm method (Permanent Methods)
   a. Fore Males:
      - Vasectomy
   b. For Females:
      - Tubectomy
      - Mini-lap operation
      - Laparoscopy.

Natural Family Planning

BOM (billing ovulation method)—that is chart your way to a happy family life.

Before explanation exhibited all the materials prepared for the general crowed to come and have a close look at each thing and create an conducive atmosphere and doubts, curiosity into there minds.

Later the second step builds the topic by simple explanation like question and answers.

Following few questions were put forward
Where the fertilization of the ovum of the woman does takes place?

It was shown in one of the chart—The fertilization of the ovum of the woman takes place in one of the ovaries of the woman. At ovulation, the egg. Ovum is released when the follicle breaks through the surface of the ovary.

What is the Ovary?

The female sex organ in which ovum cells mature and hormones are produced which influence the release of the egg cells.

When does the Human Life Begin?

Human life begins at the moment of conception/fertilization.

What is Menstruation?

It is the process of discharging blood from the uterus, usually at monthly interval from puberty to menopause.

What is Menstrual Cycle?

It is a process of ovulation and menstruation.

How Long does this Process Last Normally?

The process normally lasts 28 days. However, there can be variations from 18 to 35 days. Health conditions may affect the number of days.

What is Ovulation? Peak day?

The release of a mature ovum by an ovulation follicle during the ovulation day.

    These signs are not constant in all women. These additional signs help to pinpoint the ovulation day.

1. The most important and surest sign to determine the ovulation day is the mucus. This constant in all women.
2. Spotting of blood extends from a few hours to half-a day on the ovulation day. The woman may mistakenly that she is having two periods a month. This is normal. Nature reveals to her in red and more accurately, that her ovulation time is at hand. Women mistake it a some kind

of diseases, and approach doctor for treatment. The spotting and pain is due to the release of ovum.

3. Changes in mood from intense feeling and excitement to depression and to irritability. Husbands should be aware that their wives could have changes in their moods on the ovulation day.
4. There may be a feeling of discomfort, feeling of fullness, heaviness.
5. There may be enlargement of the breast.
6. There may be also swelling around the sexual organs.
7. There can also be a feeling of sleepiness, tiredness and aching pain.
8. Body temperature rises from ½ to 1 degree on the ovulation day. When women are instructed about these changes and signs they can easily learn to identify the ovulation day by observing. They can convincingly tell their husbands and become responsible parents by dialogue and participatory decision making regarding having or not having child.

- How to check the mucus method?
- Where/when to check the mucus?
- How to chart the menstrual flow?
- What is the importance of charting?
- Was shown by photographs chart type—the menstrual cycle-the mucus pattern of fertility and infertility
- To avoid pregnancy intercourse should be avoided during the fertile days and particularly on the peak days.

Drawbacks

A woman's menstrual cycles are not always regular. As it is irregular, it is difficult to predict the safe method—needs high degree of motivation and cooperation. Compulsory abstinence of nearly half month that is programmed sex has a high failure rate due to wrong calculations and inability to be accurate, causes anxiety.

Condom

The condom is a thin rubber sheath used by men during sex. Condom is safe and effective method of birth control. The condom is unrolled over erect penis before each act of sexual intercourse. The condom prevents the deposition of semen in the vagina. Condoms should not be reused.

Advantages

- Easily available through commercial outlets
- Easy to use
- Protects from unwanted pregnancy
- Protects against STDs and AIDS
- No side effects.

Disadvantages

- May reduce sexual pleasure
- Each time new condom should be used
- It may even slip or tear.

Withdrawal

Withdrawal is an ancient method of contraception. The male withdraws just before ejaculation and there by prevents deposition of semen in the vagina.

Intrauterine Devices (IUD)

Intrauterine devices are two types of—Medicated and nonmedicated—comes in different shapes, size, loops, spirals, coils, rings, etc. IUD contains small amount of barium sulfate to allow X-ray observation.

a. *Copper - T:* Copper - T is made of plastic material and copper wire is wrapped around the stem of the device since copper can dissolve slowly; the Copper - T may be replaced every 3 to 5 years. It has low failure rate. It is inexpensive suitable for women who are breastfeeding. It is reversible and can be removed when desired. No hospitalization is required. It is reliable method for spacing childbirth. It is not interfering with normal sex life of the wearer. IUD is a foreign body causes cellular and biochemical changes in the endometrial and uterine fluids (Arabs Middle East used for camel a small round stone into uterus. In 1909 first device made of silkworm gut. Japanese first to introduce plastic device. Today 65 million women use IUD worldwide. In that 50 million are in China alone).

b. *Lippes Loop:* It is double S-shaped plastic device made of polyethylene. It has attached threads or "tails" made of nylon. Now Copper-T is replacing the loop.

Time of Insertion: The best time for IVD insertion is between 3 and 7 days of menstrual cycle.

Side effects of IUD—Bleeding, pain, pelvic infection, uterine perforation, pregnancy, entopic pregnancy, expulsion facility after removal, cancer, mortality.

Hormonal Contraceptives

A. *Oral pills:* Oral pills contain small amounts of an estrogen and progestogen. They are effective and reversible method. They prevent pregnancy by inhibiting ovulation. They are 100% effective.

*Side effects:*Mild nausea, dizziness, headache, intermenstrual bleeding, spotting, weight gain or tender breasts.

Type of pills: Mala - N and Mala - D both contain Norgestrel and Ethinyl estradiol.

Mode of intake: A packet of oral pills contains 28 pills of which 21 are contraceptive pills and 7 are iron tablets. The first course of the pill should be started on 5th day of menstruation as day 1 - daily one tablet should be taken as indicated on packet in arrows. As packet is finished, next day new packet should be started. The pill should be taken daily at fixed time mainly at night.

B. Injectable contraceptives:

      Types: 1.   Depo - Provera (DMPA)

                    2.   Net - EN.

Both contain only progestion They are given by intramuscular injection (Net-EN every 2 months and DMPA every 3 months). The most effective methods of contraception.

C. *Subdermal implants:* Norplant is highly effective, reversible, estrogen free-contains progesterone. It is implanted subdermally.

D. *Vaginal diaphragm:* Vaginal diaphragm is a soft rubber a coiled spring rim. The vaginal diaphragm is inserted into the vagina prior to intercourse where it covers the cervix completely and prevents the spermatozoa from entering the uterus. It must remain in place for at least 6 hours after intercourse. For better effectiveness, a contraceptive jelly, cream should also be used.

Creams and Jellies

A measured quality and quantity of cream or jelly is introduced into the vagina by a special applicator just before sexual intercourse. At body temperature they melt and spread in the vagina and provide a thin film of a chemical barrier.

Rhythm Method

A week before and a week after the menses is considered as a safe period. During this period the woman is not fertile because she cannot ovulate.

Breastfeeding—lactation prolongs postpartum amenorrhea and provides some degree of protection against pregnancy.

Permanent Method

For Males

1. Vasectomy: Vasectomy or male sterilization is most effective methods of contraception. It is a permanent method of contraception. Well-suited to males having already two or more children. Done free in government hospital.

   Vasectomy is a simple, safe and a minor operative procedure that is done under local anesthesia. It involves cutting and tying off the vas deferens on each side. Blocking vas where reabsorb ion of sperms takes place. It is 100% effective.

Advantages
- Very effective method of contraception
- A very safe procedure
- Does not interrupt sex
- Does not require hospitalization.

Disadvantages—Avoid or check at least 30 ejaculation as the sperms that are in vas deferens may result in pregnancy, so use contraceptive this period to be safer side. Keep wound clean and dry, avoid cycling and lifting weight, and use T bandage after stitches removed.

For Female

1. *Tubectomy:* This is an abdominal operation in which a small piece of each fallopian tube is removed and legated. Here we showed them the poster and model we had prepared. The operation is done after giving general or spinal anesthesia. Hospitalization is required for 5 to 7 days. She is told to follow few instructions. It is a major procedure.
2. *Mini-laparoscopy operation:* It is a traditional modified laparotomy tubectomey. It is a simple procedure. It requires a small supra— pubic incision of 2 -5 to 3 cm. The tubes are cut and the ends are blocked. It is suitable for postpartum sterilization. Done at PHC level, it is less traumatic than the traditional tubectomy.
3. *Laparoscopy:* It is carried out by a team of trained surgeons/ gynecologists with a specialized instrument called laparoscope. First abdomen is filled with gas, (carbon monoxide, nitrogen or air) to push intestine away from the site of operation; one or 2 cuts are made on lower abdomen. With the laparoscope the tubes are identified and fallopian rings/or clips are applied to occlude the tubes. Short operating time, short hospital stay and small scar is characteristic feature of laparoscopy. Laparoscopic method

of tubectomy is popular. Female sterilization is 100% effective. Sexual desire is unchanged. Menstruation will continue as usual.

Winded with a theme song and short evaluation and feedback. We were happy and satisfied that large number of people came and benefited as afterwards they came in person to ask for doubts and suggestions. We advised them to go to near by PHC and get clinic services, community services, and FP services.

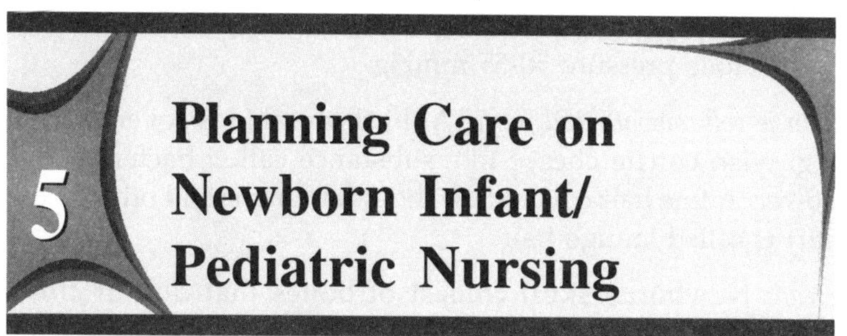

CHARACTERISTICS OF NORMAL NEWBORN

A healthy infant born of term between 38 to 42 weeks should have an average birth weight 2.7 to 3.1 kg, rise immediately following birth—establishes independent rhythmic condition and quickly adapt to the changed environment.

General Appearance

The infant lies with extremities flexed in supine position, one shoulder elevated, buttocks elevated, head turn to one side, arms extended fingers reached to midthigh level. T-activity may be increased with the stimuli.

Measurements: Head circumference—head circumference is 33-35 cm, it is 2-3 cm larger then the chest circumference.

Chest circumference is about 30.5 to 33cm. The thorax is barrel-shaped. The breathing is quiet and manly with diaphragm.

- Length on average the neonate length is 45-50 cm.
- Body weight is an average 2.5 -3.5kg, in male is 2.7- 3.5 kg; in female is 2.7-3.1kg.
- Body temperature—The normal temperature ranges between 35.5 and 37.5°C.
- Heart rate ranges from 120-140/minute.
- Respiratory rate—It ranges between 30 and 60/minute.

- Blood pressure—Systolic pressure may be 80-85 and the diastolic pressure 50-55 mmHg.

Skin is soft, smooth and puffy: At birth the skin is covered with a grayish cotrite cheese-like substance called bacteriostatic power. A fine hair covered on shoulder, thighs and other body part is called lanugo hair.

Head: Newborns skull consist of bones that do not close completely. The anterior fontanelle bounded by the partial and frontal one is diameter shaped. It is 2.5 cm long and 4 cm wide. The posterior fontanelle bounded by the occipital and partial bones is triangular shape. The widely spaced sutures indicate prematurely, budging fontanelle may suggest increased intracranial pressure and depressed fontanelle may suggest dehydration.

Eyes: Eyes are blue and gray at birth, changing to the permanent color in 3-6 month. The eyelid may be edematous for about 2 days after birth, until the kidneys eliminate the excess fluid.

Nose: Nose just after birth sneezing is common to remove the secretion from airway. Nasal flaring indicates respiratory distress.

Ear: Ear cartilage in the term infant is sufficiently formed that the ear retains its shape.

Mouth: The infant has no teeth and the sucking reflex is very active. The lips are very sensitive.

Neck: Newborns neck is short and with folds, it is in full range of motion.

Chest: Neonate breaths mainly with the diaphragm. The abdomen rises and falls at each birth. The breast may be engorged and have milky discharge because of stimulation by the maternal hormones.

Abdomen: It appears flap bowel sounds are present. On palpation it feels soft. The liver edges can be palpated

physiological immaturity of liver leads to physiologic jaundice. The umbilical cord stem contains two arteries and one vein during intra uterine period. Vein carries pure blood and arteries carries impure blood, within 7 days the umbilical stem fall down by dry necrosis process.

Genitals: In female newborn, the labia minora and clitoris are covered by labia majora. Vaginal bloody discharge may be present during first week due to abrupt crease of maternal hormones. It is known as pseudomenstruation. In male neonates the prepare is normally not retractable and the urethral opening is present at the tip. The scrotum is dark pigmented with rougher.

The first stool is passed by the infant is known as meconium and the specific gravity of the urine is low, it is straw-colored and odorless.

Extremities are in flexed position, if the extremities are extended the neonate resist and when release it will return to its previous flexed position.

CVS: Peripheral circulation is sluggish. Heart rates ranges between 120–140/minute. Cyanosis may be present soon after birth. Gradually it changes from pinkish to pale brown.

GI system: Mouth is pink, teeth are absent, and stomach has 15-30 ml of capacity. Cardiac sphincters are weak and can cause regurgitation.

Renal: Glomerular filtration rate is low and varies as fluid intake

Reproductive system: Ovaries are not functional in female babies.

Skeletal system: Hypertrophy takes place then hyperplasia.

Hematological finding: Blood volume soon after birth is about 80 ml/kg body weight.
RBC- 6-8 million/cumm
WBC- 17000/cumm
Hb- 18-20 gm%.

NEUROLOGICAL SYSTEM—REFLEXES OF NEWBORN

1. Rooting when the cheek is touched along the side of mouth the neonate ill turn his head to that side.
2. Sucking— The neonate sucks when its mouth comes in contact with a nipple or may occur as a part of a rooting response.
3. Gag reflex— Stimulation of posterior pharynx by food, suction or while passing tube cause the neonate to gag.
4. Grasp reflex— Touching palm or soles of the feet near the base of digits causes flexion of a hand and toes.
5. Moro's reflex— Moro's reflex can be elicited by holding the neonate in a supine position with the trunk just above the table and than suddenly allowing the neonate to draw backward on the level of the table. Sudden jarring or sudden lack of support case extension and abduction of extremities
6. Tonic neck reflex— The asymmetrical tonic neck reflex is elevated by placing the neonate in supine position and turning the head passively 90 degree. The flexion on the apposite extremity occur.
7. Plantar group— The plantar grasp is elicited by gently pressing the thumb into sole of a foot. The procedures flexion of the toes.
8. Doll's eyes as the head is moved to the right or left eye lays behind and do not immediately adjust to the new position of head.

Assessment of Newborn and Infant Principles of Physical Assessment

1. Begin the examination with baby on the parents lap.
2. Evaluate the chest properly you need to listen through the heartbeats.
3. The part to be examined should be completely exposed but if an apprehensive child objects hounding his cloths removed from slip your stethoscope under the shirt.
4. Using the cold stethoscope may result in a frightened and screaming child so warm the stethoscope.

ASSESSMENT OF THE NEONATE CAN BE DIVIDED INTO THREE PHASES

1. *Immediate assessment:* Apgar score system is developed by virginia's apgar in 1952. The score is based on the observation of the heart rate, respiration, muscle tone reflex, irritability and colour of the neonate. Each item is given a score of 0, 1, 2. If strongly positive, it is two and if it is negative, it is zero. The assessment starts immediately at birth, at one minute after the birth, and at five minutes after the birth. Newborn appears pink; many infants may have slight bluish-colored hands and feet due to reaction to cooler environment. While observing color of the newborn, the mucs membranes of the mouth, the conjunctiva, sole and feet is important. The muscle tone of the newborn is firm. Arms and legs are held in flexion and moving actively. Respirations are vigorous and accompanied by crying. The heartbeats are above 100 per minutes and regular. Babies normally have a score of 8-9 within first minutes after the birth. If the score is between 18-20 means newborn is easily adjusting to the extrauterine life. The score of 5-7 shows moderate difficulty of the newborn to adjust to the extrauterine life. The score od four or below four shows severe distress and may require an endotracheal intubations.

2. *Transitional assessment:* After birth, neonate tries to adjust with the environment. During the first 24 hours, changes in the vital functions such as heart rate, respiration, motor activity, color mucus production and bowel activity occur in orderly manner. This is the period of reactivity.

3. *First period of reactivity:* During the first 6-8 hours after birth, the newborn passes through the first period of reactivity. During the first 30 minutes of the period of reactivity, the neonate is alert active, cries and has strong sucking. This time is the best for breastfeeding and eye-to-eye contact. The respiratory rate may be over 60/minute. The heart rate may be over and mucus secretions are increased. Neonates heart rate, respiratory rate and temperature may be decreased.

4. Second period of reactivity starts when the neonate awakes from first sleep. That is about 6-8 hours after the birth. The period lasts for about 2-5 hours. During this period, the neonate becomes alert, active and responsive, heart rate and respiration slightly increase, gastric and respiratory secretions are increased.
5. *Physical assessment*—The order of assessment can be planned to the individual neonates. The cardiac and abdominal parts are examined when the neonate is quiet.
6. *General appearance:* Infant lies with extremities flexed in supine position. Head turns to one side, arm extended, fingers reach to midthigh level.

PLANNING CARE ON THE NORMAL NEWBORN INFANT

1. To understand the physical characteristics and the general behavior of the normal newborn infant.
2. To understand the physiology of the infant including the physiology changes which take place during the transition from intrauterine and extrauterine life.
3. To understand the major psychological aspects of the newborn infant.
4. To understand and appreciate the newborn infant as a member of the family unit.
5. To develop the ability to give professional nursing care to the newborn infant and his family.

Objectives

1. To develop skill in handling newborn infant.
2. To develop skill in performing procedures essential to the daily care of the infant.
3. To acquire knowledge of the average weight and length of the newborn infant.
4. To acquire knowledge of the normal body proportions of the infant at birth.
5. To acquire knowledge of the normal characteristics of the head of the newborn.

6. To attain an understanding of how passage through the birth canal affects the head of the newborn.
7. To acquire knowledge of the characteristic of the face and special sense organs of the newborn.
8. To acquire knowledge of the normal relationship between the various body circumstances.
9. To attain an appreciation of the significance of any deviation from normal in body measurement.
10. Learn how to care for engorged breast.
11. Care for the cord during the period of atrophic change and separation.
12. Caring for newborn genitals, maternal hormone in newborn.
13. Caring skin of the newborn.
14. Infants unstable body temperature.
15. Need for oxygen after birth.
16. Failures to establish respiration.
17. Manifestation of obstruction in the air passage.
18. Promoting lung expansion and in preventing respiratory distress.
19. Inadequate closure of fetal heart structure.
20. Establish good peripheral circulation.

KNOWLEDGE AND LEARNING ACTIVITIES

1. Picking up and handling the infant and changing his position—pick up, hold, support the baby when holding or altering position.
2. Procedures essential to the daily care of the infant-baby bath, dressing, wrapping the infant in the blanket.
3. Weighing and measuring infant.
4. Body proportion at birth compared with various development levels.
5. Demonstrating fontanel, suture and diameters of the head-observe when giving nursing care.
6. The eye color, care of the eyes immediately after birth administration of prophylactic medication at birth.

7. Taking and recording head, chest, abdomen and hip measurements and significance of any deviation from normal.
8. Breast engorgement its significance chart.
9. Observation for changing in cord stump and care of cord stump.
10. Chart characteristic of the genitals of male and female infants assisting with circumcision need.
11. Characteristic of extremities while giving nursing care.
12. Chart skin of the newborn.
13. Comprehensive physical examination a nursing care.
14. Chart demonstrating structure of the respiratory system.
15. Resuscitation of the newborn.
16. Establish respiration.
17. Observe normal breathing.
18. Chart respiratory distress.
19. Recall anatomy and physiology.
20. Observe breastfeeding, formula feeding—recording of feeding.
21. Caring for infant after elimination.
22. Demonstrate of immunization and methods of immunization in well baby clinic. Child health conference in the well baby clinic and in pediatric clinic as well as in parent education for child raring in antepartum clinic.
23. Observe daily care of the infant in field.

ASSESSING SICK INFANT
AGE 1 WEEK UP TO 2 MONTHS

1. Ask the mother what the young infant's problems are.
2. Determine if this is an initial or follow up visit for this problem.
3. Check for possible bacterial infection.
4. Has the infant had a convulsion?
5. Count the breaths, look for chest in drawing, look for nasal flaring.
6. Look for grunting, bulging fontanelle, or draining from the ear.

7. Look for umbilicus, feel for fever, skin pustules, lethargic.
8. Look at the infants movements, are they less than normal.
9. According to the sings, classify as possible serious or mild bacterial infection. According to it refer urgently to the hospital.
10. Does the infant has a diarrhea—for how long, is there a blood in the stool?
11. Look for infant's general condition such as restless, irritable, lethargic, sunken eyes.
12. Pinch the skin of the abdomen, does it go back. Assess for dehydration.
13. If infant does not have possible serious bacterial infection give fluid, frequent sips of ORS and advise mother to continue breastfeeding.

Check for Feeding Problem or Low Weight

- Ask is there any difficulty in feeding.
- Does the infant usually receive any other foods or drinks.
- Has infant any difficulty in feeding?
- If not able to feed.
- Not sucking at all.
- Thrush.
- Advise the mother how to keep the infant warm and refer to hospital.
- Check for general danger signs.
- Does the child vomit everything?
- Has the child had convulsion and does the child have cough or difficult breathing for how long?
- Does the child has fever for how long?
- If the child has measles.
- Measles with eye or mouth complications.
- Very severe febrile disease.
- Does the child have an ear problem?
- Is there ear pain, ear discharge?

- Check for malnutrition and anemia.
- Check for the child's immunization status.
- Neonatal death- a death of a live-born infant during the period that commences at birth and ends after 28 completed days after birth.
- A birth weight of less than 2500g is considered less favorable for the survival and well-being of a newborn and hence the weight of 2500 g is being used as a cut-off point. Low birth weight is a major public health problem in all developing countries. Efforts to improve birth weight should start long before the mother actually becomes pregnant.
- What is exclusive breastfeeding and how long it should be practiced?
- Why should we not give water to babies being exclusively breastfed?
- When breastfed should be stared?
- Why start BF so early?
- Can mother's milk be increased?
- What is continued BF and how long should it be given?
- When babies should be given complementary food?
- Why should not complementary food given early or late?
- What should be the type of complementary foods?
- What if mother works outside home?

PRIMARY NEWBORN CARE

- Significant reduction in newborn mortality needs to be achieved.
- What are the main causes of newborn deaths?
- Birth asphyxia, feeding difficulties, sepsis and hypothermia are the major underlying causes of preventable deaths.

Two-third of newborn deaths occur during the first week of life. Infections like pneumonia, diarrhea, tetanus, sepsis, etc are the main causes in late newborn period. Added to this poverty, illiteracy and low birth weight related causes to higher NMR.

What should be done is improve newborn care, incorporate child survival and safe motherhood program. Immunization of mother for tetanus, clean home delivery, suction and basic resuscitation at birth, prevention of infection, exclusive breast-feeding.

Special emphasis to be given to maintain of hygiene at the time of delivery in home. Cutting of umbilical cord with adequate aseptic technique, cleaning baby's mouth and pharynx, resuscitation mouth-to-mouth, weighing the baby immediately, and risk management strategies to be used.

Care and counseling of expected mothers in prenatal period with follow up during postnatal period. A community-based intervention. Detecting risk factors that are give a breath to save life be taught.

Improved survival of low birth weight babies can be achieved through educating mothers and family members on home-based neonatal care.

What is an Incubator?

Incubators are devices that help maintain the body at a desired temperature. Premature babies tend to have less fat hence lose body heat rapidly. In such situations, incubators minimize the heat loss by maintaining the immediate environment at a predecided temperature. The idea is to reduce heat loss and help premature babies gain weight.

To avoid accidents there should be a 24 × days doctors in the neonatal intensive care unit and one nurse for every two babies. Not all the incubators should be linked to a single power point, as there is fear of overload.

The electrical wiring should be independent of oxygen pipeline to avoid mishaps.

An incubator has a shelf-life of 6 to 7 years and should be replaced after that.

Incubator should be regularly serviced.

Duration of stay—The time for which a baby is kept in an incubator can vary from a couple of days of a few weeks.

The Indian manufactured incubators would cost fifty thousand and important incubators cost for two lakhs to three lacks.

How it Works?

Incubators have a baby tray enclosed in a box like the one structure made of fiberglass or acrylic, which is transparent. The heating mechanism is placed below the tray. A panel of buttons helps regulate the temperature.

In danger zone, the most common problem with incubators, noise pollution. Extensive research is being done to reduce noise inside the machines.

The baby's temperature is usually maintained at 27 to 36°C but burners are a common complaint if the incubator over heats. The newer incubators are open and binge microprocessor controlled, they do not over heat. Reich studies have shown that the electromagnetic field produced by the incubators can attack the heat rates of newborn babies.

For example, the horrific incident in which five newborns in an incubator were killed after a short circuit sparked a fire some time back it appeared in newspaper.

Regular maintenance needed to prevent such occurrence of incidents.

COMMON PROBLEMS IN NEWBORN BABY

1. Hemolytic disease of the newborn (HDN)— although it includes number of conditions, it is usually reserved for infants having as increased rate of red blood cell distinction caused by maternal isoimmunization during the first 4 weeks of life. The two most important hemolytic disease are the RH factors and A or B blood substances currently. ABO hemolytic disease is seen more frequently. It is a less severe condition and rarely caused neonatal death.
2. Isoimmunization is the development of antibodies against an antigen derived from a genetically dissimilar individual.

Routine ABO and RH typing should be done on all expectant mothers early in pregnancy to defer mine those who are type ORH negative or both.

3. *ABO incompatibility:* The major human blood type system, ABO is dependent on the presence absence of two antigenic structures. Blood types are classified on A, B,AB, and O.

4. *RH incompatibility:* The RH factor, named for the rhesus monkey in whose blood it was first observed is a thine covering of antigens that surrounds the red blood cells. If the RH antigens are present in the red blood cell, the person is RH positive. If the RH antigens are not present in red blood cell, the person in RH negative. Each person inherited three genes from each parent that is one gene from each pair. A person who is homozygous for the RH factor is termed the DD type.

5. *Hemolytic disease due to RH incompatibility:* Three-blood combination is always compatible, that is the RH factor of the blood of each parents are such that an infant mother sanitization cannot arise. It occurs when both parents are RH positive, when both parents are negative or the mother is RH positive and the father is RH negative. Erythroblastosis fetal occur that is mother RH negative and father is RH positive.

6. *Kernicterus:* Unconjugated/indirect bilirubin can pass from the plasma through the brain through the blood when there is high concentration of this substance in the blood. Indirect bilirubin exceeds 18 to 20 mg/dl. It is manifested by CNS depression or excitation. It also includes lethargy, poor sucking reflex, abnormal moro reflex, muscular rigidity, flaccidity and high pitch cry. In the final phase of it cerebral palsy, lose of ventricle gaze and high frequency nerve deafness occur results brain damage.

7. *Congenital hemolytic anemia:* The life span of an erythrocyte is about 120 days, the life span of red blood cell may be reduced due to increase and premature red blood cell destruction is taken as the only critaria for hemolytic

anemia due to increase red cell destruction but the capacity of the narrow for increased erythropoiesis is not impaired.

PREVENTION IN HEMOLYTIC DISEASE

1. *Intrauterine transfusion:* During pregnancy if the maternal antibody titer, rises and if on amino synthesis it is found that the concentration of bilirubino red pigment in the amniotic fluid is increased, an intrauterine transfusion can be given to the erythroblastic fetus.
2. *Immediate care of delivery:* At the time of delivery the goals of nursing management of erythroblastotic infants are to establish adequate ventilation and to provide oxygen as necessary neonates who have hydrops fetal is may require assisted ventilation at birth often at high inspiratory pressures.
3. *Exchange transfusion:* Brain damage become a threat to a newborn who acidemia may increase the development of kernicterus by increase the deposition of bilirubin the tissue irrespective of albumin binding status.
4. *Emotional support:* The parents of the newborn having hemolytic anemia may feel guilty about their infant's illness. This is especially true in the case of an RH incompatibility. When the mother did not receive RHOGAM after her first pregnancy. The parents can be helped to recognize that their continued parental interest is an important factor in their infants progress.

COMMON INFECTION IN NEONATES

1. Ophthalmia neonatorum may be caused by gonococci during the birth process by direct contact with infected material in the birth passage of the mother. The newborn may have redness and swelling of eyes and purulent discharge from the eyes. Culture of the eye discharge must be done to determine the organism and it as sensitivity. Instillation of choloronphencol/neomycin eyedrops used according to doctor's order.

2. Thrush/oral monoliasis: It is caused by albicans a fungal infection. It is characterized by white patches on the mucous membrane of the moth, which may bleed if an attempt is made to wipe it off. It can occurred during birth from maternal vagina infection or it can occur after birth through contact with infected hands contaminated bottle teats and contaminated hand of those who give care.

3. *Umbilical infection:* Is due to *E-coli* or staphylococci. Redness or moisture may be noticed and resulting in hepatitis and peritonitis. A discharge from umbilical lesion should be sent for a culture to determine the organism and its sensitivity.

4. Spore forming *Clostridium tetanus* through infected instrument and infected dressing used for a cord care causes tetanus neonatorum. The infant becomes restless, hypertonic, develops muscle spasm and may have opisthotonos position and unable to take feed.

5. Skin infection can vary from mild septic spots to severe impetigo or pyoderma.

6. Rubella infection is transmitted from mother to the fetus. However growth retardation, deafness may occur in the first 4th months of gestation.

7. Herpes simplex the fetal infection occurring in early pregnancy is rare. HSV is usually acquired during vaginal delivery.

8. Congenital syphilis in newborn baby passed from infected mother to fetus.

9. Cytomegalic inclusion virus disease is high in low socio-economic groups. It is transmitted through or pharyngeal secretions, urine, cervical and virginal secretion, breast milk, and blood.

10. Septicemia is a common cause of high neonatal mortality in developing countries.

11. Neonatal malaria febrile disease caused by parasite.

12. Meningitis is the inflammation of the membranes covering the brain and the spinal cord.

13. Pyelonephritis is the inflammation of the renal pelvis comes with fever, acute pain and frequency of maturation.
14. Neonatal jaundice— Is the yellow discoloration of the skin and mucous membrane due to the accumulation of bilirubin.
15. Excessive crying.
16. Abdominal distention.
17. Constipation.
18. Infective hepatitis.
19. AIDS.
20. Convulsive disorders/epilepsy.
21. Febrile convulsion.
22. Hypoglycemia.
23. Hyponatremia serum sodium level less than 139 mg/lit.
24. Hypercalcemia serum calcium greater than 12 mg/dl.
25. Hypokalemia serum potassium less than 3-5 mg/lit.
26. Hyperkalemia serum potassium more than 5.5 mg/lit.
27. Hypothermia body temperature less than 32°C.
28. Hypermagnesemia is always results from diminished urinary excretion.
29. Nerve injury, congenital malformation.
30. Spina bifida defect in closure of the vertebral column with protrusion of tissue through the bony cleft.
31. Cleft lip and cleft palate are malformation of the face that occurs. Cleft lip is results from the failure of maxillary process to fuse with the nose elevation on the frontal prominence. Cleft palate results from failure of the fusion of secondary palate with each other with the primary palate. It can be unilateral or bilateral.
32. Congenital clubfoot is a common deformity in which the foot is twisted out of its normal shape and position.
33. Esophageal atresia is failure of esophagus to form a continuous passage from the pharynx to the stomach during embryogenic development.
34. Diaphragmatic hiatus hernia is protrusion of abdominal organ through the defect in the diaphragm into the thoracic cavity.

35. Imperforated anus.
36. Intestinal obstruction.

SUMMARY

There is a difference in the anatomy and physiology of children as compared with adults. Nursing skills are specific to the care of the children and understanding children. Nurses understanding needs to develop in newborn errors of metabolism, developmental disorders, behavioral problems, pathologic conditions, sensory alteration, stress affecting family system, protection from injury, safety measures in administering drugs, reaction of family members to infants illness, infant with life-threatening events, sudden infant death syndrom, etc.

6 Health Education Model on Antenatal Care

Factors affecting education poverty, low standards of living, under developed rural areas, illiteracy, unemployment, superstitions. Education is one of the fundamental rights of all. The aim of education is to imbibe the values and live with dignity.

INTRODUCTION

Antenatal care is the systematic supervision /examination and advice of a woman during pregnancy.

Pregnancy and childbirth are special events in women's lives, and, indeed, in the lives of their families. This can be a time of great hope and joyful anticipation. It can be a time of fear, suffering and even death.

Although pregnancy is not a disease but normal physiological process, it is associated with certain risks to health and survival both for the woman and for the infant she bears.

These risks are present in every society and in every setting. In developed countries, they have been largely overcome because every pregnant woman has access to special care during pregnancy and childbirth. Such is not the case in many developing countries. Where each pregnancy represents a journey into the unknown, from which too many women never return.

The risks that woman face in bringing life into the world is not mere misfortunes. We cannot allow this to continue as

most cost-effective strategies available in the area of public health.

MMR continues to be concern across the globe, despite advances in various sectors MMR is high. Medical causes of maternal death are well known, but there is need to understand the social cause and as how to handle maternal complications.

Must focus on strengthening three things—

Universal provision of preventive quality care, identifying high-risk cases based on clinical criteria and advising them on institutional delivery and increase women's knowledge about high-risk conditions and promoting clean delivery practices at home.

Responsibility of state to provide better infrastructure and technical support and services in rural areas. Provide transport to reach urgent cases on time. In most remote areas, Dai is the only person available. Widening gap between the village and the medical system and the balance between the two is required.

With an aim to integrate traditions and technology, learn exceptional field experiences.

OBJECTIVES OF ANTENATAL CARE

1. To screen the high risk cases.
2. To maintain the physiology of pregnancy.
3. To identify anything abnormal as early as possible and get treated.
4. To provide continuing care and preventive treatment.
5. To improve the physiological status of the mother.
6. To educate the mother about the physiology of pregnancy, labor, nutrition, general hygiene and care of the baby and family planning.
7. To ensure a normal pregnancy with the delivery of healthy baby from a healthy mother.
8. Prevent complications arising out of various risk factors— additional care and watchfulness.
9. Early detection and management.

Specific objectives	Subject matter	Method of teaching	Evaluation
To explain anatomy of reproduction	Reproductive organs and its anatomy explained — female pelvis allows movement of the body during walking and running. It is adapted for child bearing, it takes the weight, protects pelvic organs.		The group understood the anatomy of female reproductive organs
Explained the importance of booking visit	Pelvic bones, the pubic born, sacrum, the coccyx, pelvic joints, pelvic ligaments, the true pelvis, the pelvic brium,cavity, outlet, false pelvis axis, types of pelvis, hormonal cycles, fertilization and early development, placenta, umbilical cord, the fetus, etc. Procedure at first visit or booking visit. The mother should register herself as soon as pregnancy is confirmed, not beyond the second missed period. She should fill in the antenatal card and history should be collected.	Lecture and discussion	
To explain the essentials of history taking	**History taking** **Personal history**—Name, age, date of first examination, address, husband's or nearest relatives name. History and circumstance of antepartum hemorrhage, eclampsia, stillbirth etc.	Lecture and discussion	Pupil understood the importance of history taking

Contd...

Contd...

Specific objectives	Subject matter	Method of teaching	Evaluation
	Age— A woman having her first pregnancy at the age of 30 or above is called elderly primy para. **Gravida**— Means pregnant woman or number of times she has been pregnant **Para**— Meaning having given birth **Parity**— Means number of times that a woman has given birth to a child, live or still, excluding abortion **Grande multigravida** is a woman who has been pregnant five times or more **Multigravida** is a woman who has previously been pregnant two or more times. She may have had an abortion or delivered a viable baby **Multipara** is a woman who has delivered two or more children **Nulligravida** is a woman who has never been pregnant now or before **Nullipara** is a woman who has never completed a pregnancy to the stage of viability. She may or may not have had an abortion previously **Primipara** is a woman who has delivered one viable child **Parturient** is a woman in labor		

Contd...

Contd...

Specific objectives	Subject matter	Method of teaching	Evaluation
	Purpura is a woman who has just given birth		
To explain the early detection and management	**Early detection and management—** 1. Poor obstetric history 2. Strikingly short stature 3. Very young maternal age/15 years 4. Prime or grand multiparity 5. Size-date discrepancy 6. Unwanted pregnancy 7. Extreme social disruption or deprivation 8. Preterm labor in previous pregnancy 9. Multiple gestation 10. Abnormal leg/presentation		Group understood the importance of early detection and management
To explain the risk factors	**Risk factors in pregnancy—** Is your height below 4 feet and 10 inches? Is your weight below 40 kgs? Are you younger than 18 years? Are you older than 30 years and this is your first pregnancy? Do you suffer from disease such as diabetes, high blood pressure, heart		Understood the risk factors

Contd...

Contd...

Specific objectives	Subject matter	Method of teaching	Evaluation
	diseases, and kidney diseases? Have you more than 3 children in 4-5 years. In your earlier pregnancy/delivery, did you have the following/ prolonged and difficult labor? Delivery through cesarean section? Abortion or miscarriage? Delivery before the 9 month? Consult your doctor and let delivery be in the hospital.		
To explain the maternity cycle	**The maternity cycle has three periods—** 1. Prenatal, antenatal or pregnancy period or period of gestation 2. Natal, intranatal, delivery or confinement 3. Postnatal or period of puerperium. Duration of pregnancy— Number of years, months Flash cards since the woman is married. **Contraceptive practice** prior to pregnancy, smoking or alcohol habits should be inquired.		Group understood the maternity cycle

Contd...

Contd...

Specific objectives	Subject matter	Method of teaching	Evaluation
	Previous history of blood transfusion, corticosteroids therapy, any drug allergy immunization history against tetanus or administration of anti-D, immunoglobulin should be inquired. History of any diseases or surgeries.		
To explain family, socio-economic history	**Family history—** Check if there is family history of hypertension, diabetes, tuberculosis, heart disease, blood disorders, any hereditary disease or twins.	Flash cards	People understood importance of family and other history taking
	Socioeconomic history— Occupation and income of the couple should be asked. Woman with low social status, there will be high chances of anemia, toxemia, prematurely, check on family planning acceptance.	Flash cards	
	Past obstetric history— This may be available if she has registered her previous pregnancy. It includes information about	Lecture	

Contd...

Contd...

Specific objectives	Subject matter	Method of teaching	Evaluation
	previous pregnancy, labor and child. Number of living children boys/girls. Health status of baby, immunization. Last child birth.		
To explain history of present pregnancy	**History of present pregnancy—** Find out the important complication in different trimesters of the present pregnancy. Any bleeding, anemia, toxemia, antepartum hemorrhage, in the last trimester. Number of previous antenatal check up if any should be noted. Ay medication or radiation exposure in early. pregnancy or any medical-surgical events during pregnancy. Any complains or disturbances in sleep, appetite, bowel habits, urination. Duration of pregnancy should be expressed in weeks. EDD— Expected date of delivery is calculated according.		

Contd...

Contd...

Specific objectives	Subject matter	Method of teaching	Evaluation
	to Naegele's Formula (EDD first day of LMP (last menstrual period plus) 9 calendar months plus 7 days or count back 3 calendar months from the first day of LMP and add 7 days to get the EDD.		
To explain physical examination	Physical examination— General— height-If height > 5 feet and shoe size>3 in first visit then the woman has normal sized pelvis Weight—Obesity can lead to increased risk of gestational diabetes. Your weight should increase in the first three months 1/2kg every month that is 1.5 kg. In the following three months 2.5kg every 15 days that is a total of 3kg. In the last three months ½ kg every week that is a total of 6kg. If you are gaining less weight or the ANC check up shows that, the size of your uterus is small. Your child	Lecture and discussion	Group understood the physical examination

Contd...

Contd...

Specific objectives	Subject matter	Method of teaching	Evaluation
	may be born with low birth weight and run risk of mortality. To gain weight should eat good nutritious food, not to carry heavy loadsrest during the day. If you gain more than 3 kg a month, then this is a sign of danger and you must consult a doctor. **TPR and BP should be checked**— Normal BP is 120/80, it should not be more than 130/90 if BP is more than this, you must consult a doctor, check it every month and make sure delivery done in hospital **Urinalysis**— It is sent for culture. Urine is tested for ketone bodies, glucose, albumin. **Blood tests-** ABO blood group and RH factored. Hemoglobin count to check for anemia. VDRL test, HIV test, rubella, sickle cell disease. **General appearance**— Obese/average/thin build. Well-nourished or malnourished. Sleep patterns. Lethargic or active		

Contd...

Contd...

Specific objectives	Subject matter	Method of teaching	Evaluation
	Face and neck— Any discharge or dryness of eyes Color of conjunctiva pallor/jaundice/anemic. Check teeth for dental carries and gum for infection. Note any crack or sores at the cornea of the mouth. Swelling of face after 6 months of pregnancy. can be serious. Look for swelling in the neck/goiter.		
Explain importance of breastfeeding	**Breasts—** Palpate for any lumps in the breast. Breast changes are observed—Increase in size of breast, areola, large blueness. Check for flat nipples or soreness/crack in nipple. **Teach about breastfeeding—** It is a fascinating fluid that supplies babies with more than just nutrition. It actively helps the newborn to avoid diseases in a variety of ways.	Lecture and discussion	People understood breastfeeding

Contd...

Contd...

Specific objectives	Subject matter	Method of teaching	Evaluation
	There is scientific evidence that some factors in human milk may induce an infants immune system to mature quickly. **Limbs—** Check for swelling of hands and ankles. Slight swelling is expected at later stage of pregnancy. Check foot end if oedema is present and report. **Bowel habits are checked—** Frequency of urination vaginal discharge, itching, offensive odor, vaginal bleeding is reported.		
Explain about diet	**Diet—** Explain abdominal examination. The diet during pregnancy should be adequate to provide for the needs of growing fetus. Maintenance of mother's health. Physical strength required during labor, successful lactation. The pregnancy diet should be light, nutritious, easily digestible and rich in protein, minerals and vitamins. Protein is essential	Lecture and discussion	People understood diet

Contd...

Contd...

Specific objectives	Subject matter	Method of teaching	Evaluation
	for the growth of the fetus. Milk, eggs, fish, vegetables, cereals, pulses etc. Iron to decrease anemia, jaggery, ragi, bajra, dark leaf vegetables, liver and kidney. Calcium to make baby's bone and teeth. Modified diet with low salt to decrease edema and high proteins for eclampsia if there is albuminuria.		
Explain abdominal examination	**Abdominal examination—** Preparation of patient— The pregnant woman should lie down on the bed during abdominal examination. She should be told to empty her bladder before the examination. She should wear loose clothes. She should be comfortable and relaxed. Privacy should be maintained. **Inspection—** The **size of the uterus** is roughly assessed. In multiple pregnancy or polyhydramnious both the		People understood abdominal examination

Contd...

Contd...

Specific objectives	Subject matter	Method of teaching	Evaluation
	length and breadth of the uterus is enlarged. In a large baby the length of the uterus increases. The **shape of the uterus** is longer than it is broad when the fetus is in longitudinal lie. If the fetus is in transverse lie, the uterus is low and broad. The shape of the abdomen in later months is egg-shaped If the abdomen is large and round with skin looking thin, suspect excessive fluid. **FHS** can be seen after 20 weeks of pregnancy. The umbilicus becomes less dimpled a pregnancy advances. The abdominal muscles are lax in multiparous woman which makes uterus sag due to pelvic contraction. Stretch marks are noted, scars may indicate abdominal surgery. **Palpation—** The hands of the nurse should be clean and warm,	Lecture and discussion	

Contd...

Contd...

Specific objectives	Subject matter	Method of teaching	Evaluation
	pads of the fingers should be used for Palpation smoothly over the abdomen, to avoid causing contractions. Estimating the period of gestation pressing gently, she moves her hand border of the fundus until she feels the curved upper border of the fundus. She notes the number of fingers between the two. Fundal height can be reassured from the symphysis pubis to the fundus of the uterus with tape measure. **Fundal palpitation—** It is carried out to know whether the fundus contain the breech or the head. Both hands are placed on the sides of the fundus, fingers helps close together and curving round the upper border of the uterus. Gentle pressure is applied to check whether it is a breech or head. An indefinite outline and soft consistency indicates the breech. If head it is distinctive in outline being hard and round. **Lateral palpation—** Hands placed at umbilicus **Pelvic palpation—** **Auscultation—**		

Contd...

Contd...

Specific objectives	Subject matter	Method of teaching	Evaluation
Explain community action for safe delivery	Ensure that all pregnant women, their family members and the community know the nearest facility where emergency care is available and make some contingency plans for transport, should an emergency arise. Problems may arise at different times during pregnancy, so the assessment for risk factors and complications must be an ongoing process. As soon as you see, any of these danger signs in a pregnant woman, rush her to a hospital. Bleeding during pregnancy, high fever during pregnancy, absent movements of her baby or abnormal presentation, severe anemia with or without breathlessness, convulsions to fits, blurring of vision or severe vomiting, bursting of water and without any pain.	Lecture and discussion	People understood community action

Contd...

Contd...

Specific objectives	Subject matter	Method of teaching	Evaluation
	Summary— visits that saves lives You must avail the following services— Register as soon as you know that you are pregnant. It is best if you register by 4 months Have 3 checkups. Have you BP checkup, have 2 tetanus toxoid injection. Have 100 tablets of iron—Anemia is a major health problem impacting on pregnancy which requires very careful management.		

Specific Objectives

1. To promote and maintain the health and nutritional status of a pregnant woman.
2. To find out high risk pregnancies and give them special care.
3. To ensure that mother receives the best available care during pregnancy.
4. To prepare the mother (physically and mentally) and material for the delivery.
5. To reduce maternal and infant morbidity and mortality.
6. To have normal, healthy and living child born.
7. To teach mother craft and responsibility of motherhood
8. To reduce the rates of babies born with low birth weight.

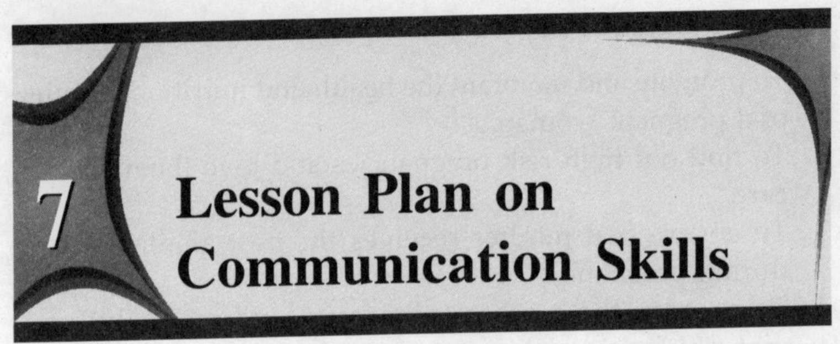

Lesson Plan on Communication Skills

- Submitted to–
- Submitted by–
- Submitted on–
- Identification data–
- Name of the subject–
- Group GNM students of–
- Place of a lecture–
- Hour–
- Topic–communication skills
- Unit–

GENERAL OBJECTIVE

To teach the students the importance of components, barriers, steps and methods of communication.

Specific Objectives

1. To explain to the students the importance of communication.
2. To make them understand the components of communication.
3. To discuss with the students steps of communication.
4. To explain to the students the barriers of communication.
5. To explain to the students methods of communication.

Time	General objectives	Specific objectives	Subject matter	Method		
5mts	To teach the students the importance, components, barriers, steps and methods of communications	To explain to the students the importance of communication	**Introduction—** Communication is defined as direct or indirect exchange of information or ideas as a means of understanding and education			
			Importance of communication— Its importance lies in exchange of information for study of problems, analysis of problem, its interpretation, comparison, problem solved. It is an educational tool, which can be used for general health population, sex, nutrition and the similar educational opportunities in health field	Lecture cum discussion	Chalk and blackboard	Under stood the importance

Contd...

Contd...

Time	General objectives	Specific objectives	Subject matter	Method	
10mts		To make them understand the compo-nents of communi-cation	**Components—** Components of communications are basically five. They are: 1. **Communicator—** One who communicates should know the need of information, to whom it pertains, its importance, detailed knowledge, method of communication and should possess art of communication. 2. **Message—** It should be clear, relevant, concise, attractive, acceptable, specific and in line with norms the community, the social and cultural norms. 3. **Channel—** The channel of communication depends upon the character of information, the time at disposal of the communicator, the seeped with which the communicate. 4. **The communicate—** The recipients his sociocultural and psychological make up	Lecture and discussion	OPH	Students under stood compo-nents of comm-unication

Contd...

Contd...

Time	General objectives	Specific objectives	Subject matter	Method		
			to grasp the message, his past experience with such information and whether it was conducive or deterrent to his behavior			
10mts		Explained the steps of communication	**Steps—** Steps involved in communication— 1. Ideation 2. Encode 3. Transmission 4. Receiving 5. Decoding 6. Action	Lecture and discussion	OHP	Students understood steps
15mts		To explain to the students the barriers of communication	**Barriers in communication—** Obstacles in communications are classified as— 1. **Physiological—** Difficulty in listening, visualizing, speaking, expressing, habits, stress and strain 2. **Psychological—** Mental tension, instability, lack of concentration, emotional disturbances, preoccupation	Lecture and discussion	Chalk and black board	Students understood barriers and of cation

Contd...

Contd...

Time	General objectives	Specific objectives	Subject matter	Method		
			3. **Environmental**— Overcrowding, poor lightening, noise, thermal discomfort, bad odors, ill maintained channels of communication. 4. **Sociocultural**— Poor knowledge of customs, practices, attitudes, habits, beliefs, language, knowledge, confidence, level of understanding.			
15mts		To explain the methods of communication to the students	**Methods of communication—** The methods of communications are— 1. **One-way communication—** that is one flow of communication in from the sender to the receiver. there is no feedback. Learning is passive. The great disadvantage is that there is no participation of the receiver in the learning process.	Lecture and dis-cussions	Chalk and black board	Students under-stood methods of com-unication

Contd...

Contd...

Time	General objectives	Specific objectives	Subject matter	Method		
			2. **Two-way communication—** In this the learner listens to the message. He may raise question to be sure he understands. He may add his own information, ideas and opinion. 3. **Verbal communication—** In this includes the use of language-whether spoken or written. 4. **Non-verbal communication—** It includes a whole range of gestures, facial expressions, smile, raising eyebrows, winking, staring, gazing, postures, body movements and even silence.			
5mts		Before winding up lecture explain the points in summary form	**Summary—** Communication can be regarded as a process by which two or more persons exchange or share ideas, facts, feelings or impressions. Communication is a complex process with many components. Barriers of	Lecture and discussion	Chalk and black board	Students under-stood the con-clusion of

Contd...

Contd...

Time	General objectives	Specific objectives	Subject matter	Method
			communication may be psychological, physiological, environmental and cultural. The methods of communication are one way, two way, verbal and nonverbal. **Bibliography—** **Assignment—** Write an assignment on methods of communication skills.	lesson

Lesson plan reveals the knowledge of teacher, her understanding of students, objectives of education, the content to be taught and her teaching ability.

The purpose of lesson planning is that it helps to select the subject matter, helps to plan activities and the preparation and test of progress; it helps the teacher to be on track, it ensures steady progress and prevents waste of time.

It helps the teacher to be orderly and systematic to check the curriculum. It helps in continuity and interconnects at the same time helps to avoid the repetition.

Teacher masters over subject matter understand student's traits, interests and background thus ensures active learning, it helps student's motivation and interest by eliminating boredom.

Lesson plan needs to be flexible and not rigid. It can be adjusted according to the situation arising in classroom.

A fresh plan should be prepared every time a teacher takes a class with latest updated information and it can be added and adjusted with changing situation. So that the objectives of the curriculum is fulfilled. So that is can serve the essentials of good teaching.

In lesson plan it should be indicated type of illustration of materials to be used. Assignments should be integrated. Evaluation done by asking questions during a class to help the teacher to understand whether the students are following the teaching with their feedback.

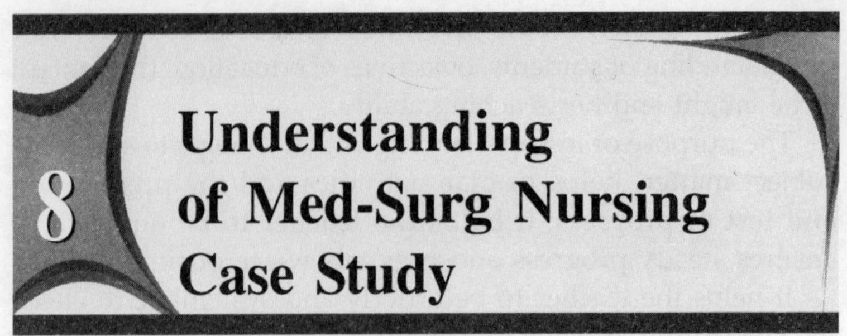

8. Understanding of Med-Surg Nursing Case Study

There are 3 distinct methods commonly used in teaching cases.
- The case study describes the life history of an individual.
- The medical case study centers about the patient, his disease and the related medical treatment.
- The nursing case study centers on the patient, his problems, his needs and nursing care.
- Both case studies attain well-rounded picture of the patient before he entered the hospital as well as facts about his illness and treatment.
- It describes all the factors relating to the development of nursing services available in the hospital.
- It presents background information of patient.
- A life history of person and whatever actions being taken.
- It helps students in learning experience.
- Here student gathers her own data on the patient, prepares her own plan of action, implements it and evaluates it under the guidance of instructor.
- Recording all the data she has gathered about the patient, as well as her own actions.
- A comprehensive study made of the individual to bring about fuller understanding of the nursing care.
- It may be a very complex case contains many problems, or it may be a simple case in which the emphasis is placed on few problems, which the students are currently studying in their classrooms.

- For example the doctor studies the patient for the purpose of diagnosis and treatment, while nurses study the disease for the purpose of deciding intelligently the best type of nursing care to be given. Here comprehensive care is given not only to patients but also to his family and his community.
- It provides an opportunity to solve nursing problems, stimulates critical reflective thinking, students learn scientific approach, it also helps to integrate their knowledge. It serves her an excellent medium to help, to develop the skills and technique needed to function well. It also provides experience to organizing and writing paper in a scientific manner.

VALUES OF THE NURSING CARE STUDY

If the care study is properly selected, directed and supervised, it provides the advantages such as—

1. It provides an opportunity for the student to solve nursing problems.
2. It stimulates the student to meet her problems by critical and reflective thinking, relating knowledge and experience from other courses to the specific condition and situation found in the patient being studied.
3. It emphasizes the fact that the patient is an individual personality and not just so many procedures or symptoms. The student learns to see patient as a person and not just as a case. Therefore care is adapted to the needs of patients.
4. The student comes to realize what an important opportunity and vital responsibility she has.
5. It points out the relationship and the cooperation of the various people interested in patients problems and welfare.
6. It acquaints the student with professional literature which has special bearing on nursing problems.
7. It enables her to record actual care given to the patient, as well as the theoretical treatment of the diseases.

8. It helps her to integrate her knowledge of the various subjects—bacteriology, pharmacology, pathology, dietetics, physiology, sociology. All are woven into one pattern, thus reinforcing her knowledge and stimulating her to search for more.

9. It contributes to the building up of a specific body of knowledge in nursing science. If the case studies are filed, they can be used for future comparisons. And when she handles similar problem, she already feels confidence to understand and treat such patient due to past case study.

The student to understand more fully the needed nursing care and not merely copying the chart.

- She must have sufficient background knowledge to solve the problem encountered.
- She needs sufficient time to study her patient as she cares for him, good morning care, sufficient materials must be available.
- She should study the patient's state of health and self help abilities, his current background, his economic level, his hobbies and interests, all these factors contribute to his welfare.
- She should study the medical aspect of his condition, patient's diagnosis and description of the diseases and the signs and symptoms as found in the patient and that she can refer the textbook and what she has learnt in classroom.
- *First part*— Information and the facts about the patient, his diseases condition and his social and personal history and how this knowledge applied in her care.
- *Second*— Giving complete nursing care to the patient— the prescribed medical orders, treatments and medicines; care given to the patient; supportive and therapeutic care, health teaching how was it met; patients likes and dislikes and special problems, nursing notes.

It is an excellent means to demonstrate her nursing skill, her scientific knowledge, her sociological and psychological insight into the problem and her skill and interpersonal relationship as a nurse with patient.

It provides self-expression in writing. Training the student to think reflectively and to judge on the basis of facts.

Clinical case assignments are made to provide the student with opportunity to learn to collect information about her patient, to determine the patients nursing needs, to make a nursing care plan and to implement, to evaluate and modify the plan as needed.

Establish nurse-patient relationship. The student to learn total and comprehensive care of patients and it takes time to get all information where she gets to know her patient and patient her nurse which leads to optimum level of health.

Nursing care plan is used to provide a guide to patient care. The written nursing plan is developed to serve guide to patient care. It is a tool; it is for today's use as well as for tomorrow's use.

All the aspects of patient's life situation, e.g. student stated that her patient could not sleep, so she gave him a narcotic.

- Was this a problem solving or was it simply the carrying out of a task?
- What did the student do to identify the cause of patient's problem?
- What nursing measures did she take to alleviate the problem?

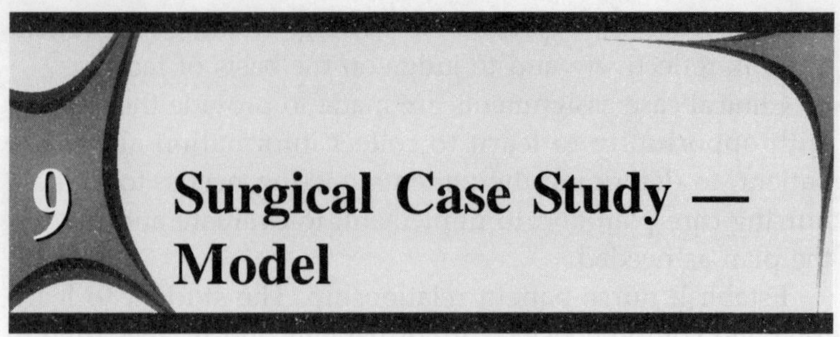

The Following Details of the Patient to be Recorded

Name of the institution–
Name of the student–
Period of posting into clinical area–
Year of course–
Submitted to–
Submitted by–
Submitted on–

Complete Data About Patient

- Identification of basic needs and problems.
- Formulation of complete nursing diagnosis.
- Planning patients needs prioritizing.
- Plan nursing actions as per objective.
- Implement nursing plan safely and accurately in given time.
- Maintain safe comfortable environment.
- Apply scientific and nursing principles.
- Meet the nutritional needs.
- Plan health instruction of family and patient.
- Record and report the data accurately.
- Evaluate the patient's response to nursing care.
- Identification data.
- Present health history.
- Past health history.

Date	Assessment	Needs/ problems	Objectives	Plan of action	Implementation	Rational	Evaluation
Pre-oprative care	The patient has knowledge deficit	Knowledge deficit related to surgery and treatment	The patient gains knowledge about surgery and treatment	Provide information about the treatment options	Provided information about the treatment options	To make patient understand and have knowledge about treatment options	Patient gain knowledge and fear and anxiety was relieved
				Give patient instructions preoperatively about wound care	Patient is instructed pre operatively about wound care	To have knowledge about surgery after operation	
				Explain the importance of treatment and hospitalization	Explained the importance of treatment and hospitalization in the presence of family	To reduce fear and anxiety about surgery	
	Patient is looking anxious.	Anxiety and fear-related hospitalization	To reduce fear and anxiety	To give psychological support to the patient	Psychological support given to patient	To give emotional support	Anxiety and fear slightly reduced

Contd...

Date	Assessment	Needs/problems	Objectives	Plan of action	Implementation	Rational	Evaluation
				Explain the procedures, types of surgery	Explain the procedures Reduced fear and anxiety	To increase confidence To relieve anxiety Divert the mind from fear	
Post-operative care	Patient is having surgical wound	To prevent infection	To assess wound for bleeding	Assessed condition of wound	To know the condition of wound	Wound was clean and no infection, swelling or bleeding	Chance of infection reduced
			To check early signs of infection	No signs of bleeding and infection	To prevent further complications		
			To do dressing with aseptic technique	Dressing done with aseptic technique	To provide healing of wound		
			Advice him to use support of	Advised support of	Enhance wound healing		

Contd...

Date	Assessment	Needs/ problems	Objectives	Plan of action	Implementation	Rational	Evaluation
				pillow while coughing and sneezing	pillow whenever cough came		
	Patient complained of pain and discomfort	Pain related to surgical incision	To reduce pain	To give comfortable position	To assess the condition	To know the condition of patient to give nursing care	Patients pain was relieved and he felt comfortable
				Give support to surgical wound	To give pain relievers as per physicians order	To provide comfortable position	
				Administered analgesic as per physicians order		To reduce pain and further complication	
	Patient is not taking food	Alteration in nutritional status less than body	Nutritional status is improved	To assess the nutritional pattern of the patient	To assessed to nutritional pattern of the patient	To improve nutritional pattern	Patient was helped to obtained

Contd...

Date	Assessment	Needs/problems	Objectives	Plan of action	Implementation	Rational	Evaluation
		requirement due to loss intake of food		Serve food as attractive manner	Served food as attractive manner	To improve the appetite	optimum nutrition
				To give high protein diet like egg, milk	High protein diet is given like egg and milk	To give strength an stamina	
				Monitor fluid intake and output fluid	Maintained fluid intake and output fluid	To maintain body fluid balance	
				To give more fluid	More fluid is given		

- Present surgical history.
- Family history.
- Personal history.
- Nutritional history.
- Socioeconomic history.
- Environmental history.
- **Head to foot examination**– General appearance, mental status, posture, vital signs, skin condition, head and face, scalp, eyes, ears, nose, mouth, neck, chest, abdomen, extremities, back, genitals and rectum, neurological tests.

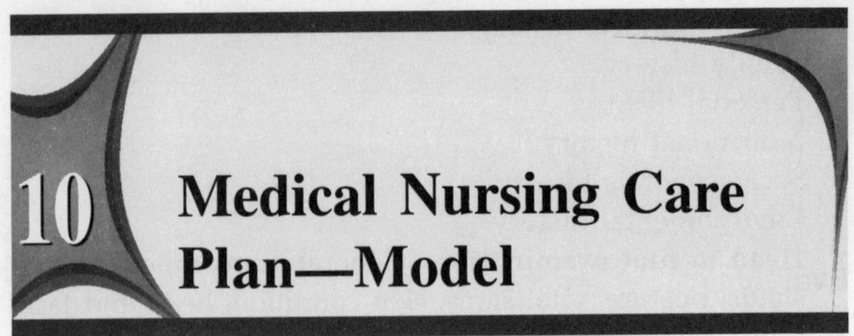

- Submitted to–
- Submitted on–
- Submitted by–
- Name of the institution–
- Name of the student–
- Period of posting clinical area–
- Year of GNM course–

Assessment

1. Collect complete data about patient.
2. Identify basic needs and problems.
3. Formulate complete nursing diagnosis.

Planning

1. Consider the patient's problems priority-wise.
2. State the objectives.
3. Plan suitable nursing action for the stated problems.
4. State rational for nursing care plan.

Implement Nursing Care

1. Complete care plan safely and accurately within a given time.
2. Maintain safe and comfortable environment for patient.
3. Apply scientific principles.

4. Meet the nutritional needs of patient as planned.
5. Give health instructions to the patient and the family.
6. Be accurate in recording and reporting patients information to the appropriate personnel.

Evaluate

1. Evaluate patients response to nursing care.
2. Reexamine and modify the patients care plan.
3. Evaluate overall performance.
4. Health instructions given.
5. Patients response to care plan.
6. Patients preparation, unit preparation, selection and organization of articles, applies of scientific principles.
7. Understand diseases thoroughly and gives comprehensive care.
8. Minimum five days care is expected.
- Student's signature.
- Teacher's signature.
- Comments by the teacher.
- Date of completion and final remark.

Identification

- Name of the patient—
- Age of the patient—
- Sex—
- Religion—
- Education—
- Occupation—
- Marital status—
- Ward number—
- Bed number—
- Date of admission—
- Surgery done—
- Consultant—
- Registration number—

- Source of information that is from patient, file, relatives, any other.
- Diagnosis— E.g. known care of hypertension with acute gastro- enteritis.
- Present health history.

A patient—E.g. A-78-years old male admitted with the complains of having loose motion with bleeding and found malena positive. He was admitted under doctor and was later diagnosed as having gastroenteritis.

Past Health History

In past health history he is under treatment for hypertension where he is taking his regular medication of his family physician.

Present Surgical History—Nil
Past Surgical History—Nil

No significance. He has not undergone a surgical operation in past or present.

Family History

- Names of family members—
- Age—
- Sex—
- Education—
- Occupation—
- Health status to be recorded—

Personal History

- Language known—
- Body built-weight-height—
- Habits-e.g. patient has bad habit of chewing tobacco, consuming alcohol, pan, supari, etc.
- Bowel and bladder regular/irregular

Nutritional History

- Types of food family take at home. Is it vegetarian, non-vegetarian like name it
- How many meals a day, etc.

Socioeconomic History

Patient belongs to middle class, high class, poor class? How many members are earning? How many of them are studying? How many educated and up to what level? How much is the income per months, by salary or business any other source, etc? How his relation with neighbor and relatives, in the village/city society around?

Environmental History

Types of house, does he live in Kachcha, rented, flat, house? How many rooms? Is there toilet present? From where do they get water? Is it well, tap of Municipality? Is there electricity in the house? Ventilation, and garbage how taken care off?

Physical Examination of Patient from Head to Feet

General appearance of patient—is he well-nourished? Is body building normal/fat/thin? Is he healthy or unhealthy? Is he active/dull? Mental status and his look/is he anxious/conscious? Is body postures and movements are normal? What is his height and weight? Normal or below normal?

- What about his vitals such as is he having temperature? How is his pulse and respiration?
- What about his blood pressure as he is known case of hypertension?
- How is his skin color, texture,? Is it pale, wrinkle? Are there any lesions, papules? How is his scalp clean? Condition of hair, dandruff, lies, hair color
- What about eyebrows normal, eyelashes/eyelids normal, conjunctiva pale, sclera normal, vision normal?

Date	Assessment	Needs/ problems	Objectives	Plan of action	Implementation	Rational	Evaluation
Day one	Patient is having alteration in his blood pressure150/ 90 mm of Hg.	Alteration in BP related to diseases condition.	To maintain normal stable BP.	To asses the condition of the patient. To check the BP every two hour and record it— Advice relatives to give salt-free diet advice the relatives activity restriction-to administer anti- hyper-tensive drugs as per physician orders.	Assess the condition of the patient Check the BP every 2 hour Advice salt restricted food advice restricted activity anti-hypertensive drugs administered as per order.	To know the condition. To know any alteration in BP. To reduce BP. To bring BP. Normal reading. To reduce pressure.	BP is slightly reduced to 130/ 90 mm of Hg.
Day one	Risk for fluid volume deficit	Alteration in fluid and electrolyte balance	To maintain electrolyte balance and diet.	Assess hydration status by examining	Assessed hydration status by examining	Helps plan care. Meet fluid needs rapidly. Regulated fluid	

Contd...

Contd...

Date	Assessment	Needs/problems	Objectives	Plan of action	Implementation	Rational	Evaluation
	related to dehydration from loose motion.	related to loose motion.		tissue turgor, mucous membranes. Assessing intake and output changes. Analyzing laboratory data—hydrate the patient avoid over hydration the patient with intravenous fluids continue fluid administration as per condition monitor intake output and specific	tissue turgor, mucous membranes. Assessing intake output changes and analyzed laboratory data's.- hydrated patient with the use of IV fluids initially- continued fluid administration with constant observation and as per need and order of physician maintain	and not to be excessive or rapid administration which may led to cerebral edema and increase ICP. For long term, fluid administration if patient condition not improved. Helps detect abnormality from normal. These are parameters to measure circulatory adequacy.	

Contd...

Contd...

Date	Assess-ment	Needs/problems	Objectives	Plan of action	Implemen-tation	Rational	Evaluation
				gravitye valuate peripheral pulses and BP at regular intervals in severe cases shomo-dynamic parameters.	intake output urine specific gravity evaluate peripheral pulses and BP at regular intervals and in severe cases homodynamic parameters.	inadequacy.	
Day one	Impaired skin integrity related to aging process, malnutrition, environ-mental	Impaired mobility related to restricted movement and debility.	To maintain personal hygiene and daily basic nursing care.	To give special attention to pressure points. Frequent change of position. Give soft smooth and	Gave special attention to pressure points Frequently changed the position Provided soft smooth	To prevent pressure sore. To prevent skin pilling. To provide smooth soft skin. To provide nourishment.	Pressure sore was prevented.

Contd...

Contd...

Date	Assessment	Needs/problems	Objectives	Plan of action	Implementation	Rational	Evaluation
	changes, poor hygiene, chronic illness, friction, soiled linen, knowledge deficit.			unwrinkled bed. Avoid prolonged exposure of the skin to hot/cold application. Provide adequate nutrition. Through cleaning of skin. Keep the skin always dry specially excessive discharge from body cavities and loose	unwrinkled bed. Avoided prolonged exposure. Nutritional need provided adequately. Cleaned skin well and kept dry specially when there was excessive discharge and wetness. Took enough protection to avoid cross infection. Gave health	To prevent friction, skin pilling, redness and bed sore. To prevent cross infection. To prevent skin diseases. To prevent from skin injury by scratching the skin. To prevent bed sore and feel comfortable and fresh.	

Contd...

Contd...

Date	Assessment	Needs/ problems	Objectives	Plan of action	Implementation	Rational	Evaluation
				motions. To take enough protection from cross infection. To give health teaching to patient and family. To cut short long nails To give active and passive exercise.	education to all cut the nails short and kept clean. Gave active and passive exercise.		
Day two	Patient is complaining pain in the abdomen.	Alteration due to discomfort and pain due to gastro-enteritis.	To relieve pain and provide comfort.	To assess the condition of patient. To assess the pain on pain scale rate. Advice patient.	To assess the condition of the patient. Advised patient not to be anxious and rest.	To reduce the level of discomfort and pain. To reduce pain.	Pain was relieved and patient felt relaxed

Contd...

Contd...

Date	Assessment	Needs/problems	Objectives	Plan of action	Implementation	Rational	Evaluation
		Altered gastro-intestinal functions due to anorexia due to diseases condition.		to relax and rest. To check vitals.	Vitals are checked. Temperature, pulse and respiration checked 2 hourly.	To know the condition of the patient.	
Day two	Patient with gastro-enteritis.		To maintain the condition under control.	Assess the ability of the patient to swallow the food before feeding starts, try with sips of water. Position the patient in upright position. Keep the suction apparatus	Assessed the ability of patient to swallow before feeding started and tried with sips of water first.Positioned the patient in an upright manner Kept the suction apparatus	To get patients cooperation. To make patient comfortable and easy to swallow. To use in case of aspiration. Patient felt happy and liked it. To prevent microorganism. To prevent chocking.	The patient improved and reduced the loose motions and melena in the stool.

Contd...

Contd...

Date	Assess-ment	Needs/problems	Objectives	Plan of action	Implementation	Rational	Evaluation
				ready. Create a conducive surrounding for pleasant meal experience. Serve food attractive way. Give month care before and after food. Encouraged small bite of food at a time. Encouraged large amount of oral fluid intake. Relieve tension. Have regular check ups to	ready bed side. Created pleasant surrounding and served meals in attractive way. Gave mouth care before and after every food. Encouraged taking a small bite of food at a time. Encouraged plenty of fluids orally. Relieved tension. Advised	To prevent secondary complications. To relieve tension. To prevent the effect of ingestion, digestion of food.	

Contd...

Contd...

Date	Assessment	Needs/problems	Objectives	Plan of action	Implementation	Rational	Evaluation
				detect early stages of problems and diseases condition.	regular medical checkups.		
Day three	Patient looks untidy. Patient has foul smell in mouth and unable to here food by mouth	Self-care deficit related to immobilization. Evidence of dryness of mouth, inflammation halitosis.	Comfort, safety and prevention of bed sore. To maintain intactmucous membrane as evidence.	Change position 2, hourly. Avoid dragging and pulling the patient while changing position. Give skin care to pressure prone areas. Avoid vigorous massage of prominences. Assess oral mucous membranes	Changed position 2, hourly. Avoided dragging and pulling the patient while changing position. Given skin care to pressure prone areas. Avoided vigorous massage of prominences bony areas.	To improve appearance and bed sore. Prevent shear force. Massage increases circulation, skin cleanliness to prevent sores. Vigorous massage causes skin excoriation over bony prominences helps plan appropriate care	Patient felt comfort and no bed sore formation. The patient maintained intake intake oral mucous membranes and no cresting found.

Contd...

Contd...

Date	Assess-ment	Needs/problems	Objectives	Plan of action	Implemen-tation	Rational	Evaluation
				for dryness, cracks, encrustations, signs of inflammation. Inspect mouth 4 hourly using flash light and tongue depressor and inspect. Cleanse and rinse mouth carefully with appropriate solution 2-4 hourly. Apply thin coat of petroleum jelly on lips after oral care.	Assessed oral mucous membranes for dryness, cracks encrustation and signs of inflammation. Insept mouth with flash light Mouth care is given by PP lotion in 1:5000 every 4 hourly. Applied thin coat of petroleum jelly on lips after oral care.	It helps to detect early complication clean mucus membranes clean, moist and free of inflammation to prevent drying cracking and encrusting of the lips	

Contd...

Contd...

Date	Assessment	Needs/problems	Objectives	Plan of action	Implementation	Rational	Evaluation
Day four.	Patient not taking food.	Nutrition lessthan body requirement related inability to eat and swallone as evidenced by weight and other nutritional parameters less than normal.	To maintain normal nutritional status.	Assess nutritional status and requirements, signs of malnutrition and emancipation noted. Administer fluids as per requirements with careful monitoring fluid intake output. Administer fluid diet in the form of juice, shake, soup, porridge, water via Ryles tube.	Assessed nutritional status. Administered IV fluids to meet nutritional needs with careful monitoring and recording intake output. Administered fluid diet in the form of juice, shake, soup, etc.	Provides base-line data to plan care. Intravenous administration meets nutritional requirements. Helps determine nutritional adequacy.	Patients nutritional imbalanced was corrected.

Contd...

Contd...

Date	Assessment	Needs/ problems	Objectives	Plan of action	Implementation	Rational	Evaluation
Day four	Inability to perform the activities of daily living.	Due to aging and diseases condition.	To maintain physical health.	To relieve anxiety. Reassure that every activity will be done with nursing assistance. To respect his self-esteem and self-confidence.	Relieved anxiety and fear. Reassured him and his self-confidence.	To relieve anxiety and fear.	Patient understood importance of daily activity.
	Isolation from social life due to poor physical health.	Due to diseases condition lead to depression.	To maintain poor physical health.	Never leave the patient alone. Arrange recreation like phone and TV facilities.	Not allowed to be left alone. Arranged recreation with TV and phone facilities.	Improve activity and meet daily needs. To reduce boredom and depression. To give physical and emotional support.	

Contd...

COMMUNITY NURSING CARE PLAN IN THE FIELD VISIT

Objective data	Nursing diagnosis	Objectives	Intervention	Rational	Evaluation
1. Mother complains of frequent loose stools since morning.	1. Alteration in bowel pattern/ diarrhea relation to GI infection.	1.STG—restore hydration status LTG—further episodes of diarrhea.	1. Assess the level of dehydration.	1. Assessment helps to manage the case.	1. The child is hydrated adequately.
2. Mother complains that the child is usually warm today.	2. Alteration in body temp/ pyrexia related to infection.	2. STG attain normal body temp LTG prevent further episodes of fever.	2. Assess TPR.	2. Appropriately reduce the body temperature. Sometimes GI infections may accompany with signs of fever.	2. Mother verbalizes the importance of cleanliness, cause, spread and prevention.
3. Child has a running nose.	3. Alteration in breathing pattern related to respiratory infection.	3. Achieved normal breathing patterns. Prevent further episodes of ARI.	3. Assess the stool color, consistency, frequency, odor.	3. Helps in maintaining hydration, as water is lost in elevated temperature.	3. Mother demonstrated the preparation of conjee

Contd...

Objective data	Nursing diagnosis	Objectives	Intervention	Rational	Evaluation
4. Child gains weight poorly.	4. Alteration in body mass due to faulty feedings practices/worm infestation/ delayed mile stoned.	4. Treat for worm infestation/ correct feeding practices.	4. Enquire on the food intake previous 24 hours. Administer ORS if mild dehydration is present. Advocate home available fluids like rice water Advice feed. Advice soft solid carbohydrate-based diet Avoid wheat and protein diets, roughen diet. Administer antibiotics. Advice cleanliness, disposal of stools, hygiene of napkins, discourage bottle feeds, health education on cause, spread and prevention. Demonstrate specific diet preparation, e.g. rice friend channa conjee, arraroot canjee, etc.	4. Correct dehydration. Organisms.	4. The child is able to breath freely following the steam inhalation.

Contd...

Objective data	*Nursing diagnosis*	*Objectives*	*Intervention*	*Rational*	*Evaluation*
5. Appearance the child looks thin and weak for the age.			Administer antipyretic and antibiotic if required. Assess the bowl pattern. Encourage mother to administer plenty of fluids, at frequent intervals and continue breast feed. Advice soft solid, non-greasy and nonoily diet. Encourage the mother to dress child with loose cotton. Not to take child to crowded place. Not to allow people with infection to handle child. Give tepid sponge, keep room, house ventilated. Health-education on causes, spread and prevention.	5. Helps in apt management and in preventing further episodes of diarrhea.	5. Child exhibits 4 to 5 episodes of infection in a year 6. Child passed worms in the stool. 7. Mother promises to monitor the weight of a child.

- Is there any ear discharge? Is hearing normal? Is there any secretion from nose or any septal deviations? How is his oral hygiene? Foul smell from mouth, discoloration of teeth, tongue pink, moist, etc.
- Is there any enlargement of lymph nodes? Range of motion, flexions, rotations normal.
- Posture, breath sound, heart sound chest.
- Abdomen observation-flatulence, distension, auscultation, tenderness, percussion, etc.
- Genitals and rectum, enlargement of prostrate gland.
- Coordination normal, reflexes, test for sensation normal.
- What types of investigations carried out for the patient?
- Blood test, urine test, stool examination, etc.

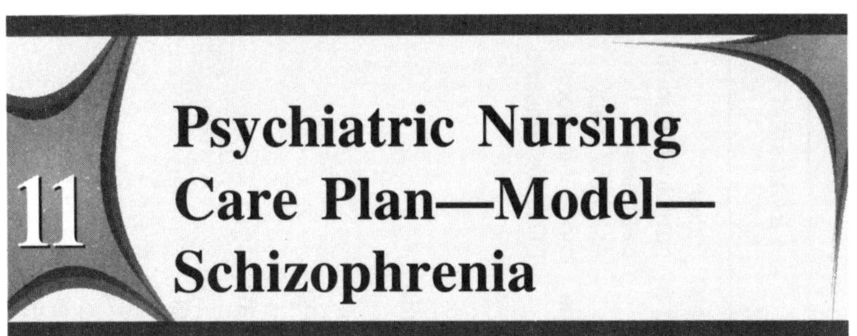

Psychiatric Nursing Care Plan—Model—Schizophrenia

Nursing care plans will vary according to an individual patients needs. Keeping the holistic care of the individual, nursing care plans.

Therapeutic Need

Physical need—Encourages personal hygiene, care of skin, improve appetite and weight, and improve the sleep pattern.

Psychological Need

Recreational activities- socialization—
Spiritual needs—
Discharge plan—

SAMPLE MODEL NURSING CARE PLAN- SCHIZOPHRENIC PATIENT

Nursing needs	Goals	Planning	Implementation	Evaluation
Therapeutic need.	To help the patient to recover. To enable the patient to learn the importance of treatment. Decrease symptoms and recover from diseases.	Plan the drug therapy with doctor and relatives. If physical therapy, ECT is to be given, it should be discussed with relatives and patients. Individual and group psychotherapy needs to be planned and given.	Give the drugs prescribed by the psychiatrist. Keep 5 R in mind. Observe for side effects Record any change in the patient after medicine. Record and report early and late side effects of antipsychotic drugs. Explain ECT therapy to the relatives. Explain to the patient he will be getting an injection for ECT. Interact with the patient at one to one level. Allow him to speak about his illness.	Patient participates in his treatment. Ask how many more injections ECT are required.
Psychological needs.	To help the patient communicate his	Plan to establish positive relationship,	Sit next to the patient when he is sad, crying	Develops trust in the nurse and

Contd...

Nursing needs	Goals	Planning	Implementation	Evaluation
To decrease disturbed thoughts.	problem effectively. Develop skill in integrating his thoughts and speaking abilities. Reduce his fantasies which may be leading to looseness of thought and autism.	help the patient develop trust in the nurse. Provide a planned opportunity for interaction.	and talk to him about his problem. Don't criticize patient. Have simple interaction and encourage him to talk.	others in communicating. Reduction in fantasies.
To reduce delusions	Help to accept reality	Plan to identify the relationship of reality and delusion.	Listen to the patients delusion and find out its relationship with his behavior.	Decrease need to use delusions.
To decrease hallucinations	To help the patient to concentrate on his tasks and care. To enable the patient to lead a productive life. Reduce his anxiety	Plan to talk to the patient to find out the reason for anxiety. Develop therapeutic relationship with patient.	Select a separate room for interaction Talk in a trustworthy and comfortable environment so that his anxiety is reduced.	Gains insight into his illness, hallucinations decrease.

Contd...

Nursing needs	Goals	Planning	Implementation	Evaluation
	Develop relationship with others.	Do not give any importance to the voices or visual objects.	Talk about all other things but not the hallucinations. Don't give any importance to the voices while interacting with the patient, refer them as so-called voices or those voices just don't bother.	
To improve communication.	To decrease anxiety associated factors while interacting to promote self.confidence To enable the patient to verbalize the problem.	Build rapport with the patient. Use an active friendly approach. Try to listen to the patient. Provide comfortable and trustworthy environment. Develop various communication techniques.	Do not ignore the patient. Initiate the conversation. Allow the patient to talk and be an active listener. Do not probe, argue or criticize. Allow silence for some time.	Develops confidence in communicating relevantly with others.

Contd...

Nursing needs	Goals	Planning	Implementation	Evaluation
To improve socialization.	To help the patient to have a sense of belongingness. To improve his self-confidence. Increase social interaction with others.	As they are withdrawn create environment for socialization so that self-confidence of patient is enhanced.	Speak in short, clear sentences. Allow him to sit with other. Take initiative to talk to the patient. Tell him to come out of bed and talk to others. Pat for his performance in the group. Tell others to come and play with him.	The patient starts making positive comments on himself. Develops feeling that he is also of some worth.
To enhance self-concept.	To help him feel worthy and competent	Help him to do most of his activities himself. Help him to remain clean.	Provide simple activities.	He feels more confident of himself.
To improve attention and judgment.	To improve the span of attention. Develop decision making ability.	Activities of such kind where attention required for a long time.	The patient may be asked to play Ludo with the nurse	Concentrates and attends to the activities, participates

Contd...

Nursing needs	Goals	Planning	Implementation	Evaluation
		Simple problems can be placed before him and asked to take decision.	Two fighting to go to bathroom at a time, he may help them in deciding.	I giving opinion on family issues.
To improve family support.	To help in adjusting a mentally ill in the family. To help family to participate in the care of patient.	Plan for the relative to be available with the patient during hospitalization Educate of the relatives about the patient is suffering	Make sure that one relative is always with the patient. Teach the relative to persuade the patient to maintain his personal hygiene, take diet, participate in day care activities and to accept the treatment.	The patient feels wanted by the family members. Looks forward to his discharge. Makes future plans with his family members.
Physical needs to Provide protection	To prevent harm t self and others. Protect from self-injury.	Provide safe environment Set limits to his behaviour Discourage impulsive acts of violence.	Avoid keeping a glass, knife, blade or any sharp instrument.	He identifies that his behavior is unacceptable and makes effort to have more self-control.

Contd...

Nursing needs	Goals	Planning	Implementation	Evaluation
To assist in personal hygiene care.	To improve his personal appearance and sense of well being. Maintain self-respect.	Ensure that he takes his bath and attends to persona hygiene, brushing, shaving. Going to toilet, bathing, changing his clothes.	Be with him. Encourage him to go and brush his teeth. Tell hi to shave, wear his own clean clothes daily him.	Starts maintaining cleanliness. Take pride in his appearance.
To improve sleep pattern.	Help him to get up fresh and active. To develop regular sleep pattern.	Try to provide a calm and comfortable environment. Have less sleep in the day time. Plan activities during the day.	Encourage to go to sleep by 10.30 P.M. Switch off the main lights Put on the bedside floor lights.	The patient has longer hours of sleep, feels less tried.
Nutritional care.	To increase his energy level. To help him develop interest in eating. Cope with any other physical stress such as infections.	Diet may be given according to the choice of the patient. Encourage and help them to eat.	Plan an adequate and balance diet. Serve food attractive manner. Persuade him to eat himself.	The patients appetite improves. Starts eating food with minimum persuasion.

Contd...

Nursing needs	Goals	Planning	Implementation	Evaluation
			Tell the relatives to taste the food, if the patient is afraid of taking it due to his delusion.	
Recreational needs	To divert the attention of the patient from his sickness To help him feel that he is recovering	Provide the activities of his interestIf the patients is too aloof, give those activities by which he can socialize.	Ask the patient what all he likes to do or his hobbies. Encourage to play badminton, carom board.	Enjoys life routine. Finds meaning in his activities.
Spiritual needs	Develop a sense of satisfaction and freedom Have a sense of recovery	Provide a place for the patient to practice his beliefs. Provide opportunities for religious activities.	Encourage him to say his daily prayer. Do not force him if he does not want to participate other religious activities. Celebrate religious functions.	Patient feels confidence of his life.
Discharge plan	To help him to lead a meaningful life in the family, in the community To enable him not to become a burden on the family and society	Help the patient to take up social and family roles whenever required.	Follow up his job is required.	The patient develops a sense of recovery.

Paranoid is commonly used term for suspicious behavior. It is replaced it with delusional/paranoid. Paranoid disorders are characterized by moderately impaired reality testing, affect and sociability.

Persons with this type personality suspect that other people will harm them. He finds people untrustworthy. He is tense, insecure, and rigid, secretive. Chronic alcoholic states and drug intoxication lead to a paranoid delusional state.

Common nursing diagnosis increased anxiety, impaired communication and interpersonal interaction, alter thought, impaired perceptions, impaired socialization, increased hostility, self-care deficit, restricted movements, sense of inadequacy and powerlessness, and family stress.

Ensure that the patient takes medicine. To enable patient to reduce his symptoms. Appreciate the need of taking treatment. Provide opportunity to clarify his doubts on his treatment. Allow the same nurse to give him medicine.

Reduce his anxiety and help him to develop trusting relationship with others. So he feels less threatened and develops interpersonal relationships. Do not put him in isolation but allow him to move freely around. Consistently try to answer his questions and doubts by using simple clear sentences.

Help him to develop insight into his problem and be more realistic. Try to provide an environment which is less suspicious. Establish a therapeutic relationship and inform change of activities.

To develop confidence and trust so that blaming others is decreased. Promote accurate perception; enable him to see things realistically. Let him express his hallucination so that gradually hears and sees an imaginary thing less frequently.

Avoid provoking or agitating questions do not laugh and answer his whys. Improve communication and socializations. Provide security. Attend nutritional needs so he takes food regularly. Ensure personal hygiene, takes bath regularly.

Improve sleep for longer hours and encourage activities during day time. To protect him from injury verbalize his hostile feelings. Observe his behavior, restrict and explain his hostile act. Check patients mental status.

Provide recreational activities and plan of activates that ill divert his mind from delusion and provide him with sense of achievement.

To provide spiritual needs and follow his routine which he gets satisfaction in life and helps to reduce a feeling of inadequacy.

Help him to adjust in family. Educate family members the importance of follow up and medicines.

Patient with Excitement

It has an excessive, activity characterized by increased motor change. Like over activity, irritability, demanding, prone to injury. Though excited, he feels worthless and useless and it is expressed with arrogance. He starts manipulating others which helps him to protect himself from failure which gives him false sense of power and control.

Due to hyperactivity there is a change in nutrition intake. Inability to sleep, change in weight, inappropriate dressing, decreased attention and concentration, impaired social functioning, impaired communication, impulsive in decision making, denial of problem.

Have a nonthreatening approach. You should remain calm and firm. Provide support, recreation and enforce limits. Accept the patient here and now, avoid arguments and canalize activities. Verbalize feelings and discouraged violent behavior. Locate the cause of disturbed behavior.

Help the patient to accept and take medicine and its effects and the need explain. As they have boundless energy, plan activity and provide adequate sleep. Improve diet and fluid intake to improve in weight. Due to exhaustion more food and fluids will be required.

Keep less furniture in the room, check the sharp instruments, glass or any other things not found near the patient. Plan to dress according to time and weather, he gradually develops judgment that he needs to be clean and adequately dressed. Pursue to attend personal hygiene.

Reduce verbal activity such as teasing, hostile, listen with concentration. Refrain himself from assault remarks and acts. Respect privacy. Observe he gets distracted too stimuli too frequent. Improve communication. See he does not use very strong words while talking to others.

Identify the method of coping with negative self-concept. Improve socialization, enable him to learn the value of life, improve the quality of life. Allow spiritual reading.

Help him in the following the instructions regarding drugs and follow up days.

Depression

It is a state associated with the mood of a personnel pessimism, hopelessness, helplessness, low self-esteem and guilt feeling?

Characterized by reduced concentration and attention, unworthiness, ideas of self-harm-suicide, disturbed sleep, diminished appetite, and pessimistic views of the future.

Originate with an experience of loss which leads to anger which he turns inward. Too much dependency leads to disappointment.

Decreased activity, apathy, loss of interest, reduces concentration, impaired communication and socialization, decrease sleep, self-care deficit.

Reduce suicidal ideation, prevent him going into stupor. Check the types of medicines keep 5 R in mind. Make observation after drug and ECT. Ensure individual and group psychotherapy; constant observation of patient.

Do not leave him alone, check the sharp instruments, glasses, rope, check if he is collecting some drugs, do not allow him to bolt doors, help him to gain insight into the seriousness of problem. Help him new ways of coping with situation.

Provide food of his choice in small quantity at a time. Pursue him to maintain personal hygiene. Balance activity rest and sleep to reduce a feeling of dependency and helplessness. Help to develop feeling of self-sufficiency, confidence that now I can manage myself. Improve communication, socialization. Reduce feeling of guilt and apathy that these types of difficulties are faced by many people. Think of alternative solution, go for group therapy.

Withdrawn behavior—Consisting of retreat from social contact and avoids an opportunity to interact with others. He tries to avoid social interaction, tries to isolate himself from others. Use an active friendly approach.

Suicide is an act or instance of taking ones life voluntarily. Causative motives—A progressive failure to adapt to stresses. Feeling of alienation or isolation, feeling of anger or hostility towards others, fantasy, reunion with a friend who died in accident, to ends the feeling of hopelessness and helplessness, a cry for help, an attempt to save face, save frustration, terminal or chronic illness, impaired through process.

It has feeling of isolation desire to kill him use to worthlessness. There is marked depression, disturbed sleep pattern, impaired communication, loss of self-esteem.

Anxiety

During the period of stress everyone goes through anxiety. An individual is able to cope up with the associated symptoms of anxiety. But when the individual is not able to do so and starts developing marked symptoms he requires help. Sometimes this basic factor of anxiety may turn into other neurotic disorders.

Anxiety is a response to an unidentified or unknown threat which may be due to unconscious conflict or insecurity. It is due to conflict, exaggerated fear, changed physiological status, lowered self-esteem, decreased family support, disturbed eating pattern, etc.

Obsessive compulsive disorder— It is a neurotic disorder, there is an obsession thoughts are ideas, images or impulses that enter the individuals mind again and again in a stereotype form. The patient is always worried about the acts he has been performing. It increases anxiety, decreased coping ability, impaired judgment, low self-esteem, need for behavior modification.

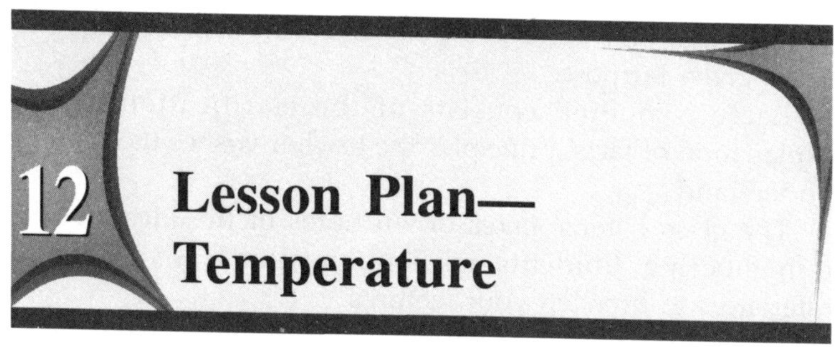

12 Lesson Plan— Temperature

INTRODUCTION

Nursing teaching helps students to acquire knowledge, understandings, skills, attitudes, values, appreciations, relevant to the area being taught- teaching and learning method highly stimulating and motivating learning. It requires intensive and active participation by the student.

Every teacher creates her own teaching method. In terms of her personality and experience, choosing and adapting available techniques. One cannot teach well by copying method which provides effective for someone else.

Teaching skill and technical competency can be developed.

Methods should be suitable to the objectives and the content of the course. Many different techniques may be used in the same class. For example a student would hardly learn to nurse a patient if she only heard lectures on the subject, as well as gaining knowledge.

Methods should be adapted to the capacity of the student; the intellectual capacity, maturity, receptiveness.

Be flexible, adjust course outline than covering so much subject matter, and academic ability of each student. Develop your own style of teaching, to suit your personality. Some are by nature humorous, outspoken, reserved, permissive, be at your best and effective.

Teaching method used be creatively and always alert, constantly to discover new ways using talents systematic self analysis and be willing to experiment with new technique to serve given purpose.

Lecture method consists of the clarification or the explanation of facts, principles the teacher wishes the class to understand.

The class listens, takes down notes of the ideas worth remembering. Students ask few questions. Give outside references to broaden your lectures.

The lecture illuminate, supplement and reinforce the topic. She may provide illustrative materials not found in the readings. Concrete examples help to provide the student with a factual basis from which to build concepts.

Know your subject and enjoy enriching, let listeners get inspired and guide them to become better person.

The goal of lecturing is communication; it is prepared before hand with objective kept clearly in mind. Lecture should provide intervals for clarification of thought, assimilation of ideas.

Teacher establishes rapport with her students.

Beginning the lecture with a review of pervious lectures, tying with present one. Use natural tone of voice and keep the students alert and address students with eye contact. The eyes have unique power to transmit the mood, language, voice, poise, vocabulary all are essential factors. The teachers fault is mirrored in the lecture. Plan carefully, emphasize, ask questions, give examples and tell interesting details which pertain the subject.

The demonstration method if of utmost important in the teaching. Is learning through observation? It projects mental image in the student's mind, which fortifies verbal knowledge and gives teacher an opportunity to evaluate the student's knowledge of a procedure.

The demonstrator should understand the entire procedure that is review before performance.

Everybody should have good view of it, running comments relative to materials used.

If live model patient is used consent.

A discussion followed, re-emphasis, questioning, recall, evaluate and summary. Still it is fresh in mind of a student should be given an opportunity to practice procedure for better learning.

Sample Class Plan

This illustrates a lecture-demonstration class in which the teacher lectures and demonstrates a procedure, and the students participate by practice and return demonstration.

Title—of the course: fundamentals of nursing.

Unit II—observation of signs and symptoms.

Time—allotted- hours.

CLASS—THE CARDINAL SYMPTOMS—TEMPERATURE

1. Objectives of the Class

a. *Central objective*—To teach the student to take body temperature by mouth and to interpret and record accurately.

b. *Teacher objectives*—
   1. To help the student to learn to read the clinical thermometer and to record temperature.
   2. To help the student realize the importance of accuracy in reading and recording the temperature.
   3. To help the student to develop a clear understanding of the principle underlying the procedure for taking body temperature by mouth.
   4. To demonstrate the technique for taking and recording mouth temperature at this hospital.

c. Student Objectives—

1. To learn the principles on which the clinical thermometer is based.
2. To learn to read a clinical thermometer and to record body temperature.
3. To appreciate the importance of accuracy in reading and recording body temperature.
4. To understand the principles underlying the procedure for taking body temperature by mouth.
5. To learn the technique for taking temperatures by mouth.

Contributory objectives	Course content	Activities
	Introduction: Yesterday we discussed cardinal symptoms with particular reference to temperature. We learned meaning and significance of body temperature and importance of taking and recording temperature carefully and accurately. Today we are going to learn how to take body temperature. We will begin by familiarizing ourselves with the instrument used for taking body temperature. (Clinical thermometer) Two scales: Fahrenheit and Centigrade.) (Necessity for knowing both).	Review by questioning. What is this instrument?
To understand how the thermometer works	Compare clinical and bath thermometer:} 1. Size	Distribute a clinical thermometer to each student.

Contd...

Contributory objectives	Course content	Activities
To appreciate the danger of breaking thermometer. To understand importance of leaving thermometer in place long enough. To understand importance of reading accurately.	2. Substance in both of thermometer: a. Bath – spirit b. Clinical – mercury, expands when heated, silver in color. 3. Range in temperature. a. Bath – 0º to 130º F. or more b. Clinical – 94º to 108º (or 110º) F 4. Time needed for thermometer to register: a. Bath – almost immediately. b. Clinical – 1 to 3 minutes. 5. Time it takes for column to drop: a. Bath – instantly b. Clinical – has to be shaken down (Bore smaller, mercury heavier 6. Markings on thermometer : a. Bath – shows change of 2º b. Clinical – shows change of 0.2º	Have one bath thermometer to show comparison. What will determine distance mercury will rise? What would happen if a clinical thermometer were placed in water over 110º F? How long does it take for bath thermometer to register? When did column of spirit drop? Use overhead projector to demonstrate thermometer readings. Have students read own thermometers, giving assistance as needed.
To be able to read the thermometer and handle it	To locate mercury: stand with back to light: roll thermometer gently back and forth between fingers. To shake down mercury: Grasp thermometer firmly at upper end; give 3 or 4 full swings that end with bulb pointing down.	Demonstrate Have students practice

Contd...

Contributory objectives	Course content	Activities
	Areas suitable for taking body temperature; must be readily assessable; must be area where thermometer can be completely surrounded by body tissue; must be well-supplied with superficial blood vessels.	
To know why thermometer must go under tongue	Commonly used areas: mouth, rectum, and axilla	Why is mouth a good area? Have students look under each other's tongues to see blood vessels?
To understand important principles underlying technique of taking temperatures? To be able to take temperature by mouth.	Important principles to keep in mind: 1. Thermometer must be clean. 2. Mercury down to 95º F. 3. Patient must not have had hot or cold food or drink for 10 minutes. 4. Place thermometer under tongue. 5. Mouth must be kept closed on thermometer for 3 full consecutive minutes. 6. Patient's cooperation is essential. 7. Check temperature if indicated.	

	Requisites :
	1. Watch
	2. TPR book
	3. Tray containing:
	  a. Thermometers in 5% phenol solution.
	  b. Container with water
		Explain and demonstrate requisites

Contd...

Contributory objectives	Course content	Activities
	c. Container with green soap solution. d. Receptacle for used wipes e. Clean wipes.	
	Procedure: Refer to procedure sheet	Demonstrate procedure, using student as patient.
To review some of the important principles	Points to remember : 1. Hold thermometer firmly and give 3 or 4 full swigs that end, with bulb pointing downward. 2. It is necessary to shake column below 95°F 3. Do not condemn a thermometer because it does not register your own temperature at normal: temperature is liable to vary a half degree above or below. Bodily temperature are also influenced by exposure to heat or cold by eating or drinking. 4. All thermometers having a correction of 0.2 at any test point. 5. To ensure correct temperature, place it as far under tongue as possible and instruct patient to close lips tightly, always allowing at least 3 minutes. 6. In cold weather, thermometers require longer time to register	Distribute TPR sheets. Refer to large drawing of TPR sheet on board and explain how to chart temperature. Have individual students read different points

Contd...

Contributory objectives	Course content	Activities
	than in warm weather because mercury is at a lower temperature when placed under the tongue. 7. Standing with back to light facilitates reading of a thermometer. 8. A clinical thermometer should not be subjected to a greater heat than 110°F, which is the full registering capacity.	
	Consider contraindication for mouth temperature and teach/learn to take temperature by rectum and axilla.	Look through pamphlet, how a thermometer is made.Practice taking temperature by mouth.

CONCLUSION

- The clinical thermometer is used in measuring body temperature and is available in both F and C scales.
- The principle on which the thermometer is constructed is the expansion of mercury when subjected to heat.
- The thermometer is made of glass and consists of a bulb containing mercury and a sterm in which the mercury rises. This column of mercury remains at the height to which it rises and must be shaken down.
- A constriction near the bulb prevents the mercury from receding and thus provides a more reliable reading.
- Bulb vary in size and shape to fit the different orifices.
- A good blood supply under the tongue and rectum.
- The body temperature should be evaluated in relation to the patients usual temperature emotional state, time of day, activity and methods used.

- Oral temperature may affect hot, cold, food, fluids, smoking, gum chewing, etc.
- Oral temperature should not be taken within 30 minutes stimulates above mentioned.
- It is wiped after removing towards the bulb with rotary motion because friction is necessary for cleanliness.
- Subnormal temperature is significant as high one as it may indicate shock, hemorrhage, or decrease body functioning. Rectal temperature most accurate because it shows inner body temperature.
- Most conscious patients are aware of the fact when there temp evaluated.
- Thermometer should not be kept longer time unnecessary.
- Nursing responsibilities—clear understanding of tools—how it used, its limitations in patients situations.
- Electronic equipment use a standard one.
- Note temperature at bedside and other special sheets.
- Rectal thermometer are lubricated to educe friction—are easily broken-handle with care.
- Place it within range of vision.

13 Ethical Aspect of Nursing and Alcoholism

INTRODUCTION

Ethical Issues in Nursing

Prolongation of life, sustenance of life, clarification of ones own values the preservation of life. The ushering of life and values that have been feasor over life time- value decision ethical dilemmas provide service with respect for human dignity, safe guarding patients right to privacy treating people equally.

1. Who should make decision for patient?
2. Do persons have an obligation to avoid activities known to cause illness that in turn, may burden society?
3. What should nurses do with confidential in information?
4. Who should decide the continuation or cessation of cancer treatment?
5. Do health care workers have right to refuse care to HIV-infected patients?
6. How can nurses serve as advocates to confused clients? Nurse have obligation to speak out.
7. Who should judge quality of life? (Nurses not to judge patients quality of life).
8. How should the decision to end/continuous mechanical ventilation be made? By patient medical team, close relatives.

9. What type of patient education is needed for informed consent to radical procedures?
10. What is the nurse's role in a 'Do not resuscitate decision' (removing life support)?
11. Is it ethical to keep dying post transplant patients?
12. What do you understand by mercy killing is it allowed?
13. Should several burnt patient, terminal cancer patient, AIDS patient be allowed to refuse treatment?
14. Should regiment mother, who engaged in substance abuse be held liable for damage of the fetus?
15. What is the nurse's role in influencing parental gender selection for hermaphrodite babies?
16. Selection of sex, clan babies, ethical.

Ethos Means Custom or Characters of a Profession and Called Code

1. *INC code of ethics for nurses:*
   - The fundamental responsibility of nurses.
   - To promote health; to restore health; to alleviate of suffering.
   - The need for nursing is universal. Unrestricted by considerations of nationality, race, creed, color, age, sex, political or social status.
2. *Nurse and people:* The nurse in providing care, promotes an environment in which the values, customs and spiritual belief of the individual are respected. The nurse holds in confidence personal information and use judgment in sharing this information.
3. *Nurses and practice:* The nurse should maintain highest standards of nursing care possible within reeling of a specific situation. The nurse uses judgment in relation to individual competence when accepting and designating responsibilities and should maintain standards of personal conduct which credit upon profession.
4. *Nurse and coworkers:* The nurse maintain a cooperative relationship with coworkers in nursing and other field.

5. *Nurse and society:* The nurses shares with other citizen the responsibility for imitating and supporting action to meet the health and social needs.

The Nurse as a Member of a Health Team

Health team consist of a group of people coordinate their particular skills in order to assist a patient or his family depends upon the needs of patient.

1. A physician who is responsible for the medical diagnosis and for determining the therapy required for the patient.
2. Number of nursing personal: The team leader/the head nurse is responsible for the delegation of duties to the members of her team and the care given to the patients.
3. Dietitians or nutritionists may be a member of who decides the diet.
4. Physiotherapist provides assistance to a patient who has musculoskeletal system disorders.
5. Occupational therapist assists patients with some important function to gain skills.
6. The paramedical technologist—lab tech, radiology tech.
7. The pharmacist prepares and dispenses medicines in the hospital and community setting.
8. The social worker assists the patients with such problems as finances.
9. Nonprofessional workers are also sometimes included in the health team.

Principles

1. Learn every ones name and never address anyone by nick name.
2. Respect every ones individuality.
3. Do not impose anything on anybody.
4. Keep emotions under control.
5. Do not be afraid to admitting ignorance.
6. Do not give and take personal; favor.

7. The teamleader should not make any excuse regarding his or her responsibility.
8. Develop habits of listening and focus attention on the problem.
9. Do not say anything that disturb others faith.
10. Be patient to others.
11. The member of a team should be loyal, honest, dependable and willing to carry out the directions of the teamleader.
12. There should be, team spirit or we feeling among members.
13. There should be mutual understanding between members.
14. There should be delegate of responsibility in a group and every member should carry out her responsibility to the satisfaction of group.
15. The relationship to the public should be decent.
16. Teach the newcamer about job, make sure that all the assignments understood.
17. The new comer of the group should feel at home.
18. Establish a good rapport among the members to achieve the aim.
19. Every member should be familiar with organization plan and the policies of the group.
20. Keep up to date with information's, avoid arguments in the group.
21. Talk in terms of other mans interest.
22. Have a smiling face.
23. Praise the lightest improvement made by others.
24. Prepare yourself mentally to accept worse.

Alcoholism

Alcohol addiction is a compulsive need for an intoxicating liquid that is from ferment Ted grain or fruit. These liquids include beer, wine, and other hard liquors.

- Person craves for alcohol cannot limit his drinking.
- He experiences withdrawal symptoms such as nausea, sweating, shaking, or anxiety.

- Craving is so great that it surpasses their ability to stop drinking.
- They need assistance to stop and to rebuild there lives.
- Alcoholic anonymous describes alcoholism as a physical condition associated with mental obsession.
- It is a chronic dependency; the personality make up of these people is weak ego and super ego. He has low self esteem and poor impulse control.
- He has decreased energy, disturbed sleep pattern, impaired judgment, increase anxiety, depression, manipulative behavior, perceptual changes, and marked withdrawal symptoms.
- What are the causes and effects of alcoholism?
- It depends on the environment and traumatic experiences in life.
- These factors include culture, family, friends, peer pressures and the way person lives.
- It can lead him to serious problems and is physically and mentally destructive.
- Currently alcohol use is involved in half of all crimes, murders, accidental deaths and suicides.
- There are many health problems associated such as brain damage, cancer, heart disease, and the diseases of the liver. Life expectancy is reduced to 10-15 years.
- Too much alcohol can destroy brain cells, leading to brain damage.
- It disturbs CNS, hindering the ability to retrieve, consolidate, and process information.
- Brain causing a blackout when totally drunk.
- It also can inflame the mouth, esophagus and stomach.
- Produce irregular heartbeats, risk of high BP, heart damage.
- Harm vision, damage sexual function, slow circulation, and water retention.
- It can also lead to skin and pancreatic disorders, weakening the bones and muscles, thus decreasing immunity.

- A large portion of alcohol is broken down in liver. Liver damage can occur leads to cirrhosis of liver.
- What to do with alcoholism?
- Have a desire to stop.
- Have the initiative to identify the cause of your alcoholic.
- Forgiveness and seek counseling to aid in healing.
- Recognize and rehabilitation center for treatment.
- Get help from family, friends and above all from you.
- To help the patient to take medicine regularly.

Reduce anxiety and depression. If the patient is found to be in an acute state of intoxication, attend to medical care and maintain vital signs. Provide adequate nutrition and maintain weight, force eating and add vitamins in the diet. Do not leave him alone; give an hot glass of milk. Rub the back and make him comfortable.

The patient may jump out of window due to disorientation, protect him from injury. Irritation, violent behavior, attacks others so observe for it. Pursued him to maintain personal hygiene. Accept him with his problem provide support of relatives and be nonjudgmental. Help the patient to identify his manipulative behavior. Enhance self-esteem, learn that he is important. Call him by name. Help him to socialize, to develop sense of support, and try out new relation. Help him to identify his hobbies.

Help him to find pleasure in life without use of alcohol. To regain insight into life to have hope and gain pleasure in life without it. Attend a follow up clinic. The patient starts his routine job and home.

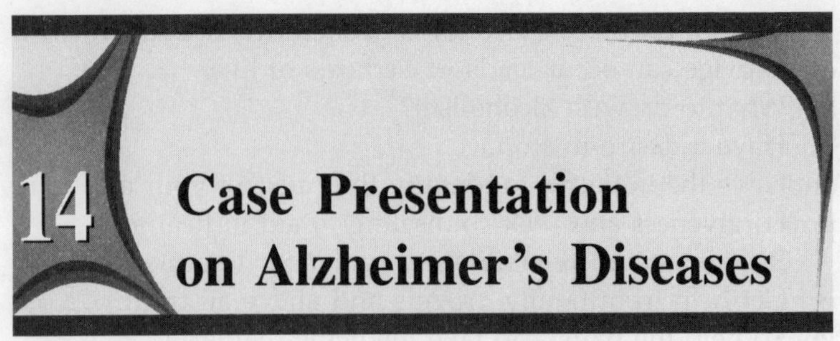

14 Case Presentation on Alzheimer's Diseases

Health education is defined as a process, which effects changes in the health practices of people and in the knowledge and attitudes selected to such changes.

INTRODUCTION

Health education is carried out in three levels such as individual, group, and public through mass media communication.

Teaching is the cheapest and most effective core of health education.

There are plenty of opportunities for health education for a nurse. The nurse have an ample opportunities to persuade people to change their behavior. Select proper group and give right education. Take up a current topic, exchange views, experience through this, and inspire people for action and to create awareness and interest. We can mould public's attitude by cheapest method of health teaching, it is the best channel to change people's unhealthy habits. Right matter put in right time with simple and direct for all to understand.

Nurse can take education to homes, schools, help, and guide every family to attain their full human rights. Therefore, she too is trained by giving the class presentation of a topic selected and presents before the students where she gains self-confidence and practice to educate people at variety of levels.

Education brings about transformation of behavior. It evolves thinking, reasoning and judgment to face the problems and challenges of life. It moulds our characters and morals. Thus awaking life dynamic and progressive creative thinking and creative awareness. It leads to integrated growth, new power and functions.

It frees us from restrains of ignorance, superstition, prejudice, blind beliefs and customs, thus leads to right knowledge, freedom and self-realization.

It is a life long process from womb to the tomb. It helps to improve quality of life. It develops the nation.

Aims of Health Education

1. To attract the audience.
2. To impress the audience.
3. To motivate audience.
4. To promote the acceptance and adaptation of the message.

Purpose of Health Education

1. To help in effective communication.
2. To minimize the barriers of language, and mis-interpretation.
3. To make the communication more lively, vivid to make more realistic.
4. To make intense effort to reach the group.
5. To give clear message on health.
6. To use creativity and inexpensive way health education.

Objectives of Health Education

1. To ensure that health is valued as an asset to the community.
2. To equipped the people with skills, knowledge and attitudes to enable them, solve their health problems by their own actions and efforts.

3. To promote the development and proper use of health services.
4. Use effective tool from selection of AV Aids available.
5. Follow the principles such as interest, participation, comprehensive, motivation, reenforcement, learning by doing, good human relationship.
6. Nurse role as a health educator, teacher, counselor, leader, messenger be realized.

Important Points to be Kept in Mind—

1. Prepare each carefully.
2. A should include teaching points, summary.
3. Never teach more than three ideas.
4. Look at the audience.
5. Do not talk too fast.
6. Include a local story, proverbs to catch interest of audience.
7. For question and answer; leave time.
8. Do not make it too long.
9. Make frequent pauses.
10. Facial expression—make audience understand that they are enjoying.
11. Remember that enthusiasm is infectious.
12. Create friendly atmosphere by greeting them and making them sit comfortably.
13. Use visual aids.
14. Up date knowledge.
15. Develop proper skill, standards.
16. Provide training to take up responsibilities and follow up.
17. Direct the capacities, attitudes, interest to desirable channels.
18. To explain memory tips.
19. To explain memory exercises that work.

INTRODUCTION OF TOPIC ALZHEIMER'S

Alzheimer's diseases affect at least 2 million and possibly as men as 5 million US residents. Ninety billion dollars spent annually for this treatment alone. Symptoms are usually subtle in onset and often progress slowly until they are obvious and divesting. And, 50–60% is genetic factor responsible for it.

It is a progressive, irreversible, degenerative, neurological disease.

In 1–10% of cases, its onset occurs in middle age. Life experiences and environmental factors also play a role in late onset.

Alzheimer's gets worse over time, and it is fatal.

Today, it is sixth leading cause of death in US.

It Destroys Brain Cells, Causing Problems—

1. With memory, thinking and behavior severe enough to affect work.
2. The patient may lose their ability to recognize familiar faces, places or objects and get lost in familiar environment.
3. The patient has difficulty in everyday activity such as handling money, using simple appliances, etc.
5. Conversation becomes difficult.
6. The ability to formulate concepts and think abstractly disappears.
7. Progression of disease intensifies symptoms.
8. The patient may wander at night.
9. Personality changes are evident.
10. Assistance is needed for eating, toileting.
11. Occasionally he may remember caregiver or family members.
12. Death occurs because of complication such as pneumonia, malnutrition or dehydration.
13. All require ongoing monitoring and vary in their level of effectiveness from patient-to-patient.

14. Duration of disease 8 to 12 years. Ist stage duration one to three years. Second stage, two to ten years.
15. It is the most common form of dementia—has no current cure, but treatments for symptoms, combined with the right services and support, can make life better for people.
16. We have learnt better to treat diseases in the last 15 years.
17. Research is in progress.

Specific Objectives of the Health Education Topic Selected

1. To introduce the topic.
2. To explain the group/class about the organ brain.
3. To explain 10 warning sings and risk factors.
4. To explain the symptoms.
5. To explain psychological stimulation and monitoring.
6. To explain importance of family support.
7. To explain diagnostic assessment.
8. To explain medical management.
9. To explain nursing management.
10. To explain importance of communication.
11. To explain physical intervention.
12. To explain psychological intervention.
13. To explain environmental intervention.
14. To explain path pathophysiology.
15. To explain clinical manifestation.
16. To explain different stages of disease progression.
17. To explain potential solution.

A sample of case presentation a student can follow:

Objectives	Methods of teaching	Subject matter	AV aids used	Evaluation
To introduce the topic	Lecture and discussion	Introduction What is dementia? What causes dementia? What are the different types of dementia? How can I tell if someone suffers from dementia? Who is most likely to suffer from dementia? How do you treat dementia? Who suffers? Dementia is a condition of the brain which causes a gradual loss of mental ability, specially loss of memory. There are changes in personality, a decline in social function, and ability to look after oneself.	Question and discussions	
To explain the organ brain	Lecture and OHP of diagram of brain showing parts and functions	Do you see the following in your loved ones? Confusion, visual-spatial disorientation, speaking difficulty progressing from anomia that is loss of ability to speak and understand, inability to calculate, delusions and hallucinations Alzheimer's and the brain- Just like the rest of our bodies, our brains change as we age. Most of us notice some slowed thinking and	Flash cards on anatomy and physiology	Group understood the brains' role in person

Contd...

Contd...

Objectives	Goals	Subject matter	AV aids used	Evaluation
		Etiology/risk factors— Increasing age, genetic disorder, head trauma, lack of education, myocardial infarction, viral infection certain factors are not been proved.		
To explain symptoms		**For such symptoms—** Consult your doctor. Get the required medical prescription. There are medicines to control the behavioral manifestations of the disease. You may be referred to psychiatric or neurologist.	Flash card	Group understood symptoms
	Discussions	**Can medicines help? Is there a cure?** Medication can help some people. However, the new drugs do not provide a cure, they have a delaying effect. There are many media reports of new wonder drugs— They usually refer to promising research. In short, there is no cure at present, but research is ongoing.	Question and sharing	Group shared experiences
To explain monitoring	Nurses intervention	**Psychological stimulation and monitoring—** Regular interaction and assurance from counselor. Rehabilitation and emotional support. Psychometric tests are undertaken periodically to understand the diseases stage.	Flash card	Group participated with discussion

Contd...

Contd...

Objectives	Methods of teaching	Subject matter	AV aids used	Evaluation
		occasionally problems remembering certain things. Serious memory loss and other major changes are sign that brain cells are failing. The brain has 100 billion neurons communicate in net work with each other. Each nerve has special job of thinking, learning, remembering, hear, smell, etc. Everything running requires coordination. In Alzheimer's part of the cells stop rerunning well. Cells lose their ability to do their job well and eventually they die.		
To explain 10 warning signs and risk factors	Lecture and discussion OHP	**10 warning signs of Alzheimer's-** 1. Memory loss 2. Difficulty performing familiar tasks 3. Problems with language 4. Disorientation to time and place 5. Poor judgment 6. Problems with abstract thinking 7. Misplace things 8. Changes in mood or behavior 9. Change in personality 10. Loss of initiative	A chart with 10 warning signs and risk factors	Group understood the warning/ risk factors

Contd...

Contd...

Objectives	Methods of teaching	Subject matter	AV aids used	Evaluation
To explain importance of family support	Family counseling	**Family support**—Assurance is important for ongoing assistance. Every member deserves to be treated with dignity. Person centered care. Social isolation and attitude damages them as much or more than the actual brain damage changing that socially built attitude to achieve benefit people with dementia.	Flash card and poster	People understood the importance
To explain diagnostic assessment	Lecture	**Diagnostic assessment—** Because there is no definitive test for DAT, the diagnosis is made by exclusion of known causes of dementia, e.g. toxic/metabolic alterations, drug side effects, cerebrovascular disease, neoplasm and infection. DAT confirmed at autopsy, postmortem examination of the brain is the only way DAT can be definitively diagnosed. The brain is viewed under the microscope for the presence of neurotic plaques and neurofibrillary tangles. Diagnostic assessments such as EEG, CT and MRI are used some times but changes in this do not appear until the later stages. Laboratory studies are currently being performed to assist in the diagnosis of it looking at beta-amyloid protein.	Flash card	People understood about the diagnostic part

Contd...

Contd...

Objectives	Methods of teaching	Subject matter	AV aids used	Evaluation
To explain medical management		**Medical management—Family can** Ask the doctor following questions when treatment started What kind of assessment will you use to determine if the drug is effective? How much time will pass before you will be able to assess the drugs effectiveness? How will you monitor for possible side effects? What effects should we watch for a home? When should we call you? Is one treatment option more likely than another to interfere with medications for other conditions is? What are the concerns with stopping one drug treatment and beginning another? At what stage of the disease would you consider it appropriate to stop using the drug? There is no cure acetylcholine are used to enhance memory and cognitive function have been disappointing. Pharmacologic therapy is aimed at treating behavior problems. Low dose antipsychotic agents can be given for agitation and confusion just before bed time.	Poster chart	Group understood medical management

Contd...

Contd...

Objectives	Methods of teaching	Subject matter	AV aids used	Evaluation
To explain nursing management		**Nursing management—** Complete history-Past medical history should be assed for previous head injury or surgery, recent falls, headache and family history of DAT. Changes in routine—Becomes agitated over small changes, apathy, social isolation, irritability as brain continues to atrophy and the limbic system becomes dysfunctional, paranoia, uses abusive language and becomes suspicious of others.	Flash card	Understood nursing management
To explain importance of communication and interaction		**Communication— Person needs effectively interacting meaningfully communication with others** It is best to speak slowly and simply with firm volume and low pitch. The tone of voice should always be calm and reassuring. They often avert their eyes, look down, back away and increase hand gesturing when they do not understand. If they get frustrated, angry or hostile, they may increase motor activity by pacing rattling door knobs, waving their arms or shaking their fists, frowning, raising their voice volume and pitch or tightening their face muscles.	Flash card	Understood effectively and meaningful interaction

Contd...

Contd...

Objectives	Methods of teaching	Subject matter	AV aids used	Evaluation
		Approach him calmly and with assurance, distract him from stressful situation or remove from situation as he may forget why he was upset. Reach out by touching, holding a hand, putting an arm around the waist or some way maintaining physical contact. Noisy breathing, constant muttering, sad or frightened facial expression, frown, tense body language could be sign of pain and discomfort. Place calendar and clock in obvious places. Past experience are shared meaningfully. Repetition is useful. Physical and environmental safety maintained. In the home, electrical devices, toxic substances, loose rugs, hot tap water, inadequate lighting and unlocked doors can be sources of injury. Wear an identification badge. Cooking should be supervised. Encourage to do as much as possible activities. Maintain his autonomy to enhance confidence and self-respect.		

Contd...

Contd...

Objectives	Methods of teaching	Subject matter	AV aids used	Evaluation
		Step by step approach for task. Anticipate elimination need and time schedule. Use clean dry clothing and bedding. Terminal stage of illness end-of-life.		
To explain physical intervention		**Physical intervention—** Obtain health history of family care giver to identify past and new health problem. Support family in following through with routine health examinations. Refer family members to physician when health problems are observed. Assess family need or adequate nutrition, hydration, exercise and rest. Help family members to be alert to signs of care giver stress.	Flash card	
To explain psychological intervention	Houe to assist family	**Psychological intervention—** Assist family to cope positively with stress. Teach stress management techniques that is relaxation, goal setting, time management, etc. Refer family to therapist when stress remains unmanageable.	Flash card	Understood psychological intervention

Contd...

Contd...

Objectives	Methods of teaching	Subject matter	AV aids used	Evaluation
		Assist family members to deal with role change and conflict. Reinforce families attempt to cope. Acknowledge family fears of being unable to continue with care giving. Refer family to support group to share with others in similar situationsIdentify family's mixed emotionsIdentify financial limitations. Help family anticipate and cope with grief process.		
To explain environmental intervention		**Environmental intervention—** Teach environmental modification. Assist family to understand symptoms related to memory loss, nature of illness, stages of disease, progression and behavior manifestation. Bridge hospital care to home care. When he leaves house and enters a potentially dangerous room alarmed, it can enable the care giver to rest at night. Keep room well-lighted.	Flash card	Understood environmental intervention

Contd...

Contd...

Objectives	Methods of teaching	Subject matter	AV aids used	Evaluation
To explain path physiology		**Path physiology—** Alios Alzheimer first described pressenile dementia in 1907. He used a new staining technique of human brain tissue to demonstrate the pathology. The changes he noted are now termed. These are abnormal proteins that accumulate in the brain. The neurotic plague is a cluster of degenerating nerve terminals, both dendrite and axonal, that contains amyloid protein. Neuritic plaques and neurofibrillary tangles are located in areas of cell loss in the brain of the patient. There are also neurotransmitter changes in the brain. A decline in cholinergic neurons in the basal nucleus leads to loss of choline acetyltrans in the neocortex and hippocampus.		
To explain clinical manifestation To explain stages of disease progression		**Clinical manifestations—** It is characterized by a relentless impairment of decision making that generally begins insidiously and can progress for a decade or so. The clinical progression of symptoms divided into difference stages-Stage 1: no impairment Stage 2: very mild decline Stage 3: mild decline	Flash card	Understood clinical management and stages of the diseases

Contd...

Contd...

Objectives	Methods of teaching	Subject matter	AV aids used	Evaluation
		Stage 4: moderate decline Stage 5: moderately severe decline Stage 6 : severe decline Stage 7: very severe decline/last stage. Memory disturbance is usually the first features. Family members or coworkers often notice the memory loss before the individual does. He demonstrates poor judgment and problem solving skills and become careless in work habit and household chores. Lack ability to adapt to new challenges. II stage- He may have language disturbances, characterized impaired word finding, speech becomes increasingly empty difficulty in using everyday objects like a toothbrush, comb, razor and utensils, serious safety problem, takes everything the mouth, etc.		
To explain final stage		**In the final stage—** Virtually all abilities are lost, including speech. Voluntary movement is minimal and the limb becomes rigid with flex or posturing. Urinary and fecal incontinence is frequent. The person has lost all ability for self-care.	Flash card	Group understood final stage and potential solution

Contd...

Contd...

Objectives	Methods of teaching	Subject matter	AV aids used	Evaluation
To explain potential solution		**Potential solution—** Monitor personal comfort. Check pain, hunger, thirst, constipation, full bladder, fatigue, infections and skin irritation. Maintain a comfortable room temperature. Avoid arguments and confrontations. Redirect persons attention, try to remain flexible, patient and supportive. Create calm atmosphere, avoid noise, glare. Provide adequate rest. Get safety locks, remove guns.		
To explain the memory tips		**Memory tips—** Be in the moment- Focus on learning, do not focus on the past or worry about the future while you are learning. Do not multitask, as you create a brain drain when you focus on more than one activity. Create a learning environment. If you are a visual learner, create tool visuals that help you retain information. Same way if you are auditory learner purchase tape recorder to repeat instruction. Use all your senses as drawing and writing, talk to another person.		Group understood memory tips given

Contd...

Contd...

Objectives	Methods of teaching	Subject matter	AV aids used	Evaluation
		Use mnemonic devices—Visual images, colorful three dimensional, it is easier to remember. Organize, e.g. writing address in address books, telephone numbers in telephone book, making a grocery list, keeping the keys in the hook meant for it, etc. Retain a positive attitude— If you constantly tell yourself and others that you have a bad memory, this action actually hampers the ability to your brain to remember.		
To explain memory exercise that work		**Memory exercises that work—** Pay attention develop a habit of actively paying attention can save much frustration. For example you have had to search for a car keys, been in doubt as to whether or not you took your morning medication correctly, or found yourself in the room wondering-pay attention-stop-look-listen. It takes no more than a second to say I a putting the key in my pocket. **Rehearse-repeat-** For example you are in the shower and get an idea you wish to discuss with your spouse. You cannot make a note, and you do not want that great new idea to slip away. What to do? You repeat to yourself your idea to talk to your spouse.		Group understood tips of exercise that work

Contd...

Contd...

Objectives	Methods of teaching	Subject matter	AV aids used	Evaluation
		Get organized— List your medication needs by time and place to be taken. Medications taken before, with or after meals are usually stored in the kitchen. Keep all emergency information as visible as you can. For example appointment books, memo pads, clock radios, timers, take-away-spots near door, in the hall, on the refrigerator.		

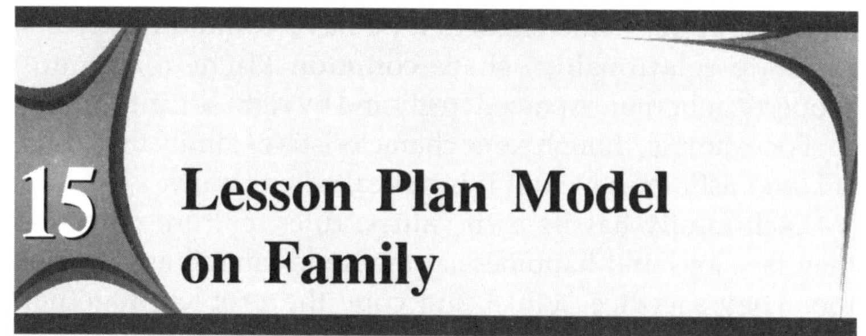

15. Lesson Plan Model on Family

Introduction

What does family mean to you?
Why do you feel like returning home at the end of the day or after holidays or picnic?
What is the importance of family life?
Why some homes fail?
What is the secret that binds the family together?
What causes stress in family?
What are the causes of breakage of family?
How to prevent conflicts, disputes, fights in the family?
What is the foundation of family is it love or is it money and property?
What are the feelings of children who do not have there own family?
What keeps family united?
What is the aim and characteristic of good family?
What are the advantages and disadvantages of living in the family?
What is the nuclear family? What is joint family?
What are the aims and objectives of family?
What are the functions of family?

Family is a universal phenomenon. Family is oldest institution found in all corners of the world. Family is related with blood and live under same shelter, they have common interests, intimate relationship, share common kitchen, common property, inheritance passed freely and by right security, union.

For example, though same characteristic of family the hostel, jail, and ashram have but it is not called as family.

Each family has its own values, rules, culture. Together they face joys and happiness at the same time illness, sorrow too. They sacrifice, adjust and cope the problem together. Money is managed in common and all needs are meet.

One person's welfare affects the other. They are interdependent. There entire life revolves around it. Home is a place of our dream. It is alive with countless warm memories. People spent whole life to make a home. In moment of advisory family supports each other and keeps emotional bond.

Mother is the center of home. Love, care, sharing is the foundation of family life. Emotional bond, accountability, commitment is mark. Every child born in family grows and receives protection. What is the family mean can be known to the one who does not have his own family. Result children get maladjusted and weak family building collapses. All need family even animals and birds have some kind of nest and family.

In family, child should be always wanted and eagerly awaited and not an unexpected guest. Parent's responsibility is to plan a child. Parents have to set example, live honestly, have integrity. Little things mean a lot to each other.

Spend quality time with your family. Talk, play and spend time with each other. It is in the homes of the family the secret of nation lies. Family is the backbone, of our social system happy family produces happy children, and happy children make happy nation. Family provides social security and stability.

Children quite often learn many things from their parents even though the hereditarily factor possess much influence children are made up by the way their environment moulds them. Parents have a leading role in the make up of all the character of every individual child. Child observes every minute movement of his parents. They often enact like parents. So, it should be taken care of and set an example to them.

Types of Family

- Nuclear where couple with children, e.g. hum do, humare do
- Joint family
- Family size—two child norm
- Polygamy—is more than one wife
- Polyandry—more than one husband
- Monogamy—universal one to one; patriarchal father is the head of family and matriarchal mother is the head of the family.

Joint family—Motto 'union is strength'—grandparents, grand children, uncle, aunts live together.

Joint family consists of a number of married couples and their children who live together in the same household. All of them are related by blood. All the property held in common. There is a common family purpose to which all the family income goes and from where all the expenditures are met. The male head shares his power and shares responsibilities. It provides economic and social security to the old and helpless and the unemployed. It pools income for the welfare of the young.

Today due to modernization, urbanization joint families are disappearing. It is common in the west. A household where representatives of three generations. It occurs when young couples unable to find separate housing accommodation and continue to live with their parents and have their own children. There is a sharing of responsibilities, greater economic and social security, old are safe, and security to helpless and unemployed. It pools its income to help the young through education. Division of labor, the head male has sole duty to earn a living. Family is a bridge. Common culture, eating pattern, dressing, language, behavior pattern, and attitudes are transmitted through family. Inheritance of property, ownership and handed down, passed from one generation to another. Teaching young, values, beliefs, codes of conduct.

Functions of Family

- Residence—family provide clean decent home to its members
- Division of labor
- Socialization
- Economic function
- Child raring
- Personality formation, care of the depended adults
- Improve the quality of life.

There is Sharing of Responsibilities

- Reproduction and procreation of children
- Each family experience its own dynamical of formation growth, maturation and dissolution, effects of sudden shift in economic status, migration, uprooting, disasters, physical change or incapacity of a family member.

Family Budgeting

To meet the basic needs of family budget is needed. When the prices are constantly increasing, it becomes difficult. An amount of expenditure for a few months will show how much money is spent under which head and where exactly one could economize. Keeping a calculation of the amount of expenditure with savings.

Advantages—It improves the life status. Helps family to do expense according to family income. It helps to develop habit of savings and helps them to lead a happy life. It helps in time of crisis and sickness. It encourages wise spending. it makes a person to make proper use of money.

- If there is a surplus that is income is more than expenditure so saving can be done. If it is deficit difficult to save.
- So family income and expenditure has to be coordinated and balanced.
- Cut down recurrent expenditure like the money spent on servants.
- Grow your own vegetables like a kitchen garden.
- Cut down the expenditure on electricity.
- Proper selection of articles, e.g. cotton clothes are more expensive to wash and wear.
- Do not postpone repairs. A stitch in time saves nine.
- Change personal habits, e.g. if rice is costly use wheat.
- Do not borrow money.
- Take a part-time job to support family income.
- Cut luxuries, cultural, recreational wants.

The Secret of Happiness and Health Lies in the Homes of People

Withstand stress and strain. The family acts as a placenta. The family is like a shock absorber to the stress and strains of life that illness and death emotional upsets, worry, anxiety, economic insecurity attain mental equilibrium and strive to maintain a stable relationship with other people.

Familial susceptibility to disease such as hemophilia, diabetes and color blindness, diabetes and mental illness are known to run through families. Schizophrenia, psychoneurosis, communicable diseases are known to spread rapidly in families because of the common environment which the family members share. Congenital malformation higher in blood relationship marriages.

Broken family—parents separated or death has occurred 'mental deprivation' the home life is utterly unsatisfactory, backwardness, poverty, illness, emotional instability, character defects and marital disharmony.

LESSON PLAN ON FAMILY

Identification Data

Name of the teacher—
Subject—
Topic—
Unit—
Date and time of class—
Place—
Group of students—
Methods of teaching—lecture and demonstration.
Teaching aids—black board and chalk, OHP.
Previous knowledge of the student—

GENERAL OBJECTIVES

Students will understand the definition, characters, family cycle, and interdependence of family members and basic needs of the family.

SPECIFIC OBJECTIVE

1. To introduce the topic with introduction
2. To explain the definition of the family
3. To explain the characteristic of the family
4. To explain types of family
5. To explain aims and objectives of family
6. To make them understand the family cycle
7. To explain the interdependence of family members
8. To make them understand the basic needs of the family.

IMPORTANT POINT WHILE PLANNING LESSON PLAIN

The students have short span of attention, every 5-10 minutes they are distracted either physically or mentally-hence it is teachers' responsibility to make their teaching innovative and interesting.

Time	General objectives	Specific objectives	Subject matter	Method of teaching	AV aids used	Evaluation
5 minutes	Students should know the definition.	To explain the definition of family.	**Subject matter** Family is known as a primary group, social institution, and basic unit of the society and a key association of the human society. The family fulfils basic needs of the society. Family is the cradle of the socialization of the child. **Definition**-MacIver and Page defined family as a group defined by a sex relationship sufficiently precise and enduring to provide for the procreation and upbringing of children.	Lecture cum discussion.	Black-board and chalk.	Students understood the definition of family.
15 minutes	To explain the charac-teristic of the family.		*Characteristics* **Important characteristics are—** 1. There is mating relationship between the husband and wife in a family. 2. There is a form of marriage in the family such as monogamy, polygamy and polyandry. 3. There is also a system of family such as father, mother, brothers, sisters, etc. in the family. 1. In the family there is economic provision 2. A common home or household is also a characteristic of the family'	Lecture and discussion	Black board and chalk with OHP.	Students understood the charac-teristic of family.

Contd..

Contd..

Time	General objectives	Specific objectives	Subject matter	Method of teaching	AV aids used	Evaluation
			3. There is a close interaction between members of the family. 4. The maintenance of a culture is also characteristic of the family.			
10 minutes	To explain the inter-dependence of family members		**Interdependence of family members—** The family is a group which has close, direct, durable and personal interaction between its members. In the personal relations are very essential for the healthy development of the family. These interpersonal relations can also be termed as familial and marital communications.	Lecture and discussions.	Black-board and chalk	Students understood the inter-dependence of family members
15 minutes	To make them under-stand the basic needs of the family		There are different types of interpersonal relations, they are— 1. Husband-wife relations 2. Parents-child relations 3. Sibling relations the modern family is known as democratic family, that is the authority is the family is shared by parents and children.	Lecture and discussion.	Black board and chalk	The students understood the basic needs of the family

Contd..

Contd..

Time	General objectives	Specific objectives	Subject matter	Method of teaching	AV aids used	Evaluation
10 minutes			**Basic needs of the family** The family is the most vital social institutions as it fulfils very important functions such as— 1. Affection 2. Sex 3. Procreation 4. Upbringing of the children 5. Religion 6. Socialization.			
10 minutes	To make them under-stand the family cycle		**Family cycle**— The family cycle or the various stages in the development of family from culture to culture the cycles are— 1. Birth 2. Child 3. Adolescence 4. Youth 5. Adulthood 6. Old agemaclver and page have indicated the following:	Lecture and discussion	Black board and chalk	The students understood the family cycle

Contd..

Contd..

Time	General objectives	Specific objectives	Subject matter	Method of teaching	AV aids used	Evaluation
			1. The formative prenuptial cycle. This stage is marked by an increasing intimacy of man and woman. 2. The nuptial stage—This is the stage before the arrival of the offspring. It involves the living together of mates, creating the environment of the home, evolving new experiences 3. The childbearing stage—The third stage fulfils the family proper linking the parents to another by the vital links of their own children, the fruits of sex union. 4. The maturing stage—This final stage emerges when the biological functions of the parents have been fulfilled and the children no longer require parental care.			

SELF-INTROSPECTION FOR TEACHER

- Do I know the underlying educational philosophy of the school in which I am teaching?
- Do I view the students experience in the clinical setting as a part of the nursing course?
- Do I have good rapport with my student?
- Do I know my students, there individual abilities, interests and needs?
- Are my students motivated and stimulated for study?
- Do I provide a variety of teaching learning activities such as well thought out problem assignment?
- Do I provide valid, reliable and objective examination to measure the outcome of my course?
- Do I participate in research and study at every opportunity so that I can help to improve teaching in schools of nursing?

Effective teacher avoiding useless repetition and irrelevant material during lectures.

Respect for the students maturity and sense of responsibility.

Through knowledge of her subject matter, each class period clear, distinct, pleasant and well-modulated voice assignments clear and concise.

Teacher should be well-balanced personality, professionally well-groomed, self confident and attractive in her personal appearance, never too busy to give a few words of encouragement.

Updates topics and trends, teaching at the level of the group.

Students can be modeled constructively with guidance. Example is mighty tool of teaching, students often imitate their teacher character send modeled and slowly formed to guide its destinies. A portion of what so learned today is forgotten tomorrow. What remains and becomes the basis for the further growth is that which enters into the total personality, change in habits and attitudes, reconstituting ideals, enlarging interests wake in them new dreams, new vision.

Thus, the teacher and nursing must be deeply concerned about the attitude and the values that her students develop as well as the clinical knowledge and the technical skills that they acquire. Motivating studies to archive desirable goal.

Dare not to enter it unless you love it. Student centered teaching, patient catered instruction. Advances have influenced nursing. What are the nursing needs for society? How can they best be met? What should be objectives for the educational programs in nursing be? What then is nursing? Is nursing a personal service given to meet the needs of a person who cannot meet the needs of a person who cannot meet his own health needs? Is it technical focusing on the carrying out? Complex procedures accurately and correctly? Are there different levels of functioning such as professional nursing, technical nursing, vocational nursing?

Tendency to blames students for the ills of the teacher. If the teacher cannot inspire and motivate them that teacher has failed.

Plan her program in logical sequence towards desired goal. Read all books available to you on the subject; draw your knowledge and experience. Jot down suitable facts under headings, check and recheck them to be up to date as well practical. Be prepared to answer there questions. Explain difficult points in various ways.

16

Psychiatric Nursing

The foundation of mental health is laid in early childhood period. The various factors contribute to mental health—good physical health is the basis of mental health. Proper functioning of all the system of the body is essential. Individuals who suffer from physical defects, deformities, disabilities and chronic incurable diseases fall in easily victim of mental illness. When the basic needs of an individual are not satisfied, there is a tendency of frustration lead to maladjustment. Worry and tension sap vitality and upset mental balance. Certain organic diseases of the body such as hypertension and coronary heart diseases occur. Insecurity due to poverty, ignorance, disturbed home condition. Basic needs of an individual are satisfied where there is love and understanding.

Mental illness was always associated with ignorance, superstitions and fears. Mentally ill patient went through a lot of torture and problems for lack of development in the field of psychiatry.

In 19th century understanding of the human behavior came. 20th century introduction of the physical forms of treatment followed. 4th decade pharmacology for the mentally ill was introduced.

Historical Periods

- The period of persecution 1552 BC-1400 AD.
- The period of segregation 1545 AD-1800 AD

- The humanitarian period 1745 AD-1826 AD
- Beginning of scientific attitude 1796-1878 AD
- The period of prevention 1885 AD-1960 AD.

Period of Persecution

- Treatment of patient depended on men's various superstitious beliefs.
- It was thought that sounds and motion are the factors of illness and health.
- Black spirit, harmful white magic.
- Patients were thrown out of society and beaten up by the people. They were tortured and left on their own. No nursing was required that time.

Period of Segregation

- In this period they were put separately in asylums, to prevent the mentally ill patients from staying into streets.
- In England, Bethlehem asylum founded first time.
- The government only founded these hospitals but patients do not had adequate condition.
- Only aim is to segregate patients from the general public.

Humanitarian Period

- More and more asylums were set up.
- Physicians got interested in working on mentally illness.
- In this period nomination of nurses were made.
- In 1773, in the United State, mentally ill patients were admitted to Pennsylvania hospital but hospencial training were given onto them who looked after mentally ill patients.

Beginning of Scientific Attitude

Jean Martin Charcot practiced hypnotism. Sigmund Freud 1856-1939 founder of psychoanalysis believed that hypnotism for causing psychic tension.

- 1860 first Florence Nightingale nursing school was opened at St. Thomas Hospital in London.
- 1873 there was first psychiatric nurse for America graduated from the New England Hospital for women and children. She organized service and education program in various state hospitals of all illness and helped to organize the first school of nursing to prepare nurses to care for mental illness.

Period of Prevention

- 1950 the national association of mental health.
- 1953 wide publicity was given to mental illness.
- 1960 first worldwide mental health year celebrated.
- 1950 paplais classic book, interpersonal relation is nursing provided.
- Nurses were prepared to identify special behavior and nursing procedure of psychiatric patients for patients care.
- 1946 the health survey committee recommended psychiatric nursing also.
- 1980 elective subject of psychiatric nursing for the students of diploma in nursing education introduced.
- Scope—need of psychiatric nursing is felt at all level of graduate courses and specialist on this is psychiatric nursing is expected to teach and participate in clinical field and do the research work in psychiatric nursing.

General Principles of Psychiatric Nursing

Patient is accepted exactly as he is— It means setting of positive behavior to respect him as an individual human being. Acceptance is expressed in following ways—

1. Be nonjudgmental patients behavior is not judged, he is not punished for his undesired behavior.
2. Interest in patient as a person is shown- study the patients behavior, spend time with patient, be aware of patients likes and dislikes.

3. Recognize and reflect on feelings which the patient may express—The nurse observes the feelings of the patient and acts accordingly.
4. Talk with a purpose—The nurse talks around the patients needs, interests and wants.
5. The nurse listens to the patient.
6. Permit patient to express strongly held feelings-encourage him to express his strong covered up negative feelings without punishment in verbal or sympathetic manner. The nurse makes him comfortable as much as possible.

When a person not able to adjust and adapt to his society he is said to be unhealthy. It requires balance between the body, mind, and spirit to cope difficulties of life successfully.

Healthy person is well-adjusted to himself; he knows his strength and weakness, is able to trust others and develops ability to give and to receive. He takes his daily responsibilities well. He has awareness of self, capacity to work, knowledge of their strength and limitations, has self-respect and acceptable behavior.

When this gets disturbed an illness occurs which comes as a symptom like depression, feeling of anxiety, severe mood changes, withdrawal results.

Nurse needs to focus on the strength of a patient. Develop therapeutic relationship with patient. Be nonjudgmental, be active listener and show professional interest. Avoid physical and verbal restrains and be consistent in behavior accept patient as a holistic human being, which leads towards the road to recovery.

Appropriate reinforcement helps in correcting maladaptive learning. There are various types of stressors, which may cause emotional and physiological disturbances in an individual. Nursing practice based on theoretical concepts. Psychiatric nursing promotes mental health, prevent and cope with mental illness and to find a meaning in life experiences. Nurse helps the patient to understand his problems. She also assists the patient to understand his problem realistically. Helps to find out new alternatives for his problem, helps to adopt new patterns of behavior, understand the problems, overcome barriers, assist patient, encourage patient, and evaluates progress towards goals. Ability to observe and interpret observation ability to guide.

Nurse's role is significant to protect the patient from drug-induced complications, modifying environment causing maladaptive behavior, vigilant observation and watchfulness attitude of kind firmness.

Self-understanding as a therapeutic tool—the nurse has to understand herself. Patient's behavior may produce fear or anxiety in the nurse, nurse has to understand why she is anxious or frightened.

A nurse can understand herself better by exchange personal experience freely with her colleagues. Discuss her personal reaction with an experienced person. Participates in group conferences in patient care

For the security of patient, consistency used, where patient feels he can depend on people working in the ward. Consistency maintained in all nurses an in all shifts. Attempts to win patients liking.

Reassurance to be Given in a Subtle and Acceptable Manner

The nurse gives reassurance to patient to build up confidence. Pay attention to the matters that are important to the patient. Listen to personal problems without showing surprised. Think with him to solve it.

Patient's behavior is changed through emotional experience, not by rational interpretation. Patient's behavior is based on emotional needs. Corrective emotional experience can bring behavior change. Help the patient to feel emotionally secure.

Unnecessary increase in patient's anxiety should be avoided-by avoiding careless conversation within patients hearing. Use of professional terms indiscriminately.

- Calling attention to patient's defects
- Lack of proper orientation
- Talking against patients psychotic ideas

Observation done of mentally ill to understand 'why' of behavior.

Maintain realistic nurse-patient relationship. Verbal and physical force must be avoided if possible. Nursing care centered on patient as a person not on control of symptoms. Routine and procedures should be explained at patient's level of understanding. Many procedures can be modified but basic principles remain unchanged.

Role of a nurse is to identify emotional problems and early symptoms of mental illness. Help the family members to cope up with stress. Arrange counselling services for the individual and family with mental conflict disturbance parent-child relationship. Hospital-based and community based rehabilitation is important to achieve goal. Educate the family to receive and treat the patient as an individual. Create motivation for regular follow up and for compliance with drug therapy.

Nurse's role in community mental health service— Case finding:
- Assessment of the individual needs
- Establishment of the therapeutic environment
- Consultation with the other professionals
- Advice participation with the health team including individual and family
- Involvement and coordination with health services
- Education of groups within the community.

Qualities of a Psychiatric Nurse

Acceptance of patient as he is, as a sick person, regardless of color, creed or behavior more abnormal the behavior greater the acceptance.

- She requires developing capacity to understand his needs.
- She must be trustful, honest, reliable and with scientific background.
- Able to act responsibly, that mentally ill persons are human beings.
- Use her intellectual capacity to maintain regular standards of education.
- Professional with good manners and good appearance.

Functions

- Meeting physical and mental needs
- Assessing with modalities
- Providing safe and comfortable environment
- Helping the patient to be in touch with reality
- Protecting the patient from effects of abnormal behavior
- Helping to improve social skills
- Educating the patient to cope with crisis situations
- Helping the patient and family rehabilitate with disabilities
- Cooperating with the members of health care team and promoting health status of the patient.

Expression of feelings within the safe limits, objectivity must be maintained. Use specific therapeutic and problem solving techniques.

- Maintain define boundaries. Encourage patient to become independent.
- Observe what is happening to patient and overall his condition.
- Assess anxiety level.
- Identify patient's expectations of a therapeutic relationship
- Increase his self-esteem.

Provide Supportive Environment for Change

- Accept the patient as having value and worth as an individual.
- Maintain relationship on professional level.

- Interactions with the patient can be carried out on his intellectual, emotional and developmental levels so that patient is able to express feeling more effectively.

The principle based on the concept that each individual has an intrinsic worth and dignity and has potentialities to grow.

Convey the feeling of being loved and cared. Do not judge behavior as good, bad, right, spent time with him, recognize and reflect on feelings which he may express.

Encourage patient to talk, let him express his anxiety, hatred, anger to release bottled up emotions and strong feelings unexpressed.

The nurse makes the observation of non verbal communication, e.g. dry lips. The nurse repeats what the patient is saying. The nurse highlights the feelings which helps to clarify his doubts. The nurse tries to link the events and feelings or persons together.

The nurse questions the patient to get information.

She is aware the causes of failure in communication.

She knows when to speak and when to be silence. Ability to proceed at the patients speed.

Psychotherapy is a form of treatment of an emotional nature in which a trained person deliberately establishes a professional relationship by removing, modifying, and reducing disturbed behavior. Help to resolved inner conflicts, develop coping mechanism, overcome handicap, reduce discomfort and improve social functioning and develop ability to perform appropriately.

Types of individual psychotherapy's are psychoanalysis, hypnosis, abreaction, reality therapy, uncovering, environmental modification, reassurance.

Bringing modification in the personality, suppressed impulses and memories, internal conflicts and childhood trauma. The therapist remains passive, no direct advice given to therapy used.

Hypnosis is a deep trace-like sleep. It is induced in a patient by suggestions of relaxations and concentrating attention on a single object.

Abreaction is a therapeutic technique in which the patient talks about repressed emotions, unconscious conflicts by reviving and reliving painful experiences that have been buried in the conscious.

Reality therapy which is focuses on the present behavior and development of a patient's ability to cope with the stresses of reality and take greater responsibility for the fulfillment of his needs. Have a realistic behavior and teaches him better ways to meet his needs in real world. The stressed on that past cannot be changed take right action of the present.

Uncovering/insight technique is needed to break through the repressed conflicts and traumatic experience to the surface. It helps the person to gain an insight.

All these techniques are aimed to correct situational problem, symptom rectification, strengthening existing defenses, prevention of emotional breakdown and teaching new coping skills.

Techniques Used

Ventilation where free expression of feelings or emotions. Patient is encouraged to take freely where he unburdened his feelings by sharing himself.

- To improve the well being of patient their living conditions are changed by environmental manipulation.
- Persuasion and reeducation person learns more effective ways of dealing with problems and relationship.
- Reassurance is a way of supporting him and encouraging him that there is a possibilities of improvement.
- Suggestion patient is given different ideas, views, ways and adjustment brings improvement.
- All this helps the patient and gives him an opportunity to release tension. It helps him gain an insight into his problem and provides an opportunity to practice new skills. It reinforces an appropriate behavior.

Modifying maladaptive behavior with adaptive behavior through new learning experience.

In cognitive therapy helps patient to change his thoughts, feelings and behavior about himself and gradually patient is able to adapt to certain behavior with guidance and help.

To handle the difficulties in a constructive manner there are other therapy too, e.g. marital therapy, family therapy, transactional analysis, group therapy, etc.

ECT—Electroconvulsive therapy is a painless form of electric therapy. A small amount of electric current is applied for a fraction of a second through electrodes placed on the temple region. This immediately produces tonic and clonic stages of convulsions (amount of current average 110 volts for 0.1-1.0 second) usually 6-10 ECT are given, it is spaced, that maximum in a week 3 ECT are given.

Indicated in major severe depression, with suicidal risk, with stupor, with melancholia, with psychotic textures, no improvement with drugs, where drugs are contraindicated schizophrenic and not responding to other treatment, early morning insomnia, lack of concentration, anorexia, etc.

ECT is contraindicated in tumor, hematoma, subarachnoid hemorrhage, resent myocardial infarction, severe hypertension, severe pulmonary diseases, thrombophlebitis, bleeding disorder, etc.

Nowdays these surgeries are not done— Psychosurgery is a surgical intervention, to severe fibers connecting one part of brain with other to destroy brain tissue with the intent of modifying behavior, mood, thoughts disturbances which do not respond to psychotropic drugs, ECT, and psychosocial therapies.

Indicated in chronic depression, chronic severe obsessive compulsive disorder, chronic severe anxiety, severe pathological, uncontrolled aggressive of all these conditions fail to other above therapy.

Surgeries done are techniques of stereotactic methods used. So, that the lesions is precise and less side effects.

- Biomedical leukotomy
- Rostra leukotomy
- Prefrontal leukotomy.

The lesions are made by electrocoagulation freezing thermocoagulation, ultrasonic methods or laser.

Procedures

1. Sterestaeit subcaudate taxonomy—A large subcaudate lesion is produced for severe depression and anxiety.
2. Steraactic limbic leukotomy—A small subcaudate lesion is made also in cingulated bundle bone for schizophrenia.
3. Angulotomy done for pathological uncontrolled aggression failure to adjust, laughing without any reason, getting violent, being abusive, doubting that somebody is going to kill, putting poison in the food, treating clothes, destroying articles, hitting, trying to injury self and other, not orientated to time, place, and person.

If a piece of rubber is overused beyond the limits of its elasticity, it is spoiled. Similarly, if an individual suffers anxiety frequently due to stressful situation and is not able to cope with it, he is maladjusted.

Nurses need to understand terms frequently used in clinical areas.

Disorders of adult personality and behavior are due to individuals lifestyle, e.g. personality disorder, habit and impulse disorders, general identity disorders and disorders associated with sexual development.

Mental disorders are incomplete development of intellectual abilities and adaptive behavior.

Some start during childhood due to poor development of central nervous system ego disorders of speech and language, disorders of scholastic skills, disorders of motor function.

Behavior and emotional disorder in childhood and adolescence.

Organic mental disorders due to brain disease, e.g. delirium, dementia, hallucination, mood disorders, personality disorder, etc.

Delirium is a type of psychosis, acute in onset, characterized by disturbances of consciousness, memory, intelligent and alteration. It is due to impaired of brain tissue function.

Etiology

Predisposing Factors

Preexisting brain damage or dementia, aging, alcohol, cerebral lesion, chronic medical illness, postoperative period, history of head injury, etc.

Metabolic Causes

Hypoxia, carbon dioxide narcosis, hypoglycemia, hepatic encephalopathy, cardiac failed, cardiac arrest, metabolic acidosis, alkalosis, hypovolemic shock, high fever, severe anemia.

Early diagnosis help prompt treatment, clinical lab test, EEG, serum chemistry, blood sugar, renal function test, thyroid function test, ECG, X-ray skull, brain scan, MRI, lumbar puncture, urine analysis, etc.

- Management identifies the cause and immediate correction done.
- Supportive medical and nursing care.
- Nutritional needs are met.
- Input out put chart maintained diseases condition controlled by medication.
- Occupational therapy may be given.
- Recreational therapy given' rehabilitation done with the help of special worker.

Schizophrenia is a group of mental illness characterized mainly by disturbance in thinking, affect perception, psychomotor activity and behavior which leads to disorganization of the personality of an individual.

Nursing Management

Patient may be incoherent—
- Call by name
- Establish a nurse-patient relationship.
- Accept the patient as he is, use nonauthoritative language and simple short words to inform the pain of treatment.

Patient has Hallucination and Delusion

- Be firm and remain with the patient
- Be watchful in noting patient's hallucination
- Build a positive and trusting relationship with patient
- Use warm, honest tactful approach, do not argue with patient
- Encourage patient to express his thoughts, fear and problems
- Divert his mind to reality
- Increase social relationship
- Help the patient to modify perception of self.

Patient may have Evident Behavior

- Observe the patient for clues that he is getting out of control
- Observe rising of anger-verbal and nonverbal behaviour
- Note his response to staff
- Maintain calm manner, be supportive and stay with patient
- Never close the room, always keeps a watch on the patient
- Avoid joking, laughing and whispering in front of patient
- Provide a safe, secure and therapeutic environment.

Nutritional Needs

- Provide a balance diet according to the choices of patient
- Weekly weight chart maintained
- Adequate fluid and electrolytes maintained.

Rest and Sleep.

Personal hygiene is maintained. Clean clothes and nursing care provided.

Occupational therapy—teach social skill, recreational activity like music, gardening.

Dopamine is a chemical released in the brain and increased production of this dopamine transmits the nerve impulses to the brainstem faster than normal results in strange thoughts.

Early observation and prevention of complications is duty of a nurse. A close observation especially when antipsychotic agents are just started.

Encourage patient to take medicine at bed time due to sedative effect.

Plan and provide comprehensive nursing care to patient with common psychiatric disorders. Select plan develop skills, observe the various signs and symptoms, report and record.

Mental Status Examination (MSE)

Identification data—
Name—
Age—
Sex—
Bed no—
Ward no—
Marital status—
Religion—
Literacy—
Occupation—
Income—
Language—
Nationality—
Address—
Date of admission—
Duration of stay—
Final diagnosis—

General Appearance and Behavior to be Noted

Physique and body build and physical appearance, i.e. height, weight and appearance
Personal hygiene maintained or poor
Dress according to seasons, clean
Hair combed or uncombed
Posture
Looks—Comfortable/uncomfortable
Facial expression—Sad looking, or happy
Any gestures
Talk and speech—
Speech coherent, irrelevant, tone of voice, spontaneous or hesitant
Gait and posture—Normal or abnormal
Motor activity—Increased or decreased
Frighten or worrie—d or happy
Appears—Calm, quiet, sad looking
Orientate to time, place, person
Memory intact
Perception, illusion
Judgment logical.

Past history of illness—
Medical/surgical illness—
Psychiatric illness—
Personal history—infancy, childhood-adolescence; adulthood, late maturity, family history.

When was symptoms first noticed, was it sudden or gradual, was there weight loss, weight gain, modification in sleep, appetite, personal hygiene, what is his educational level, his status in his working place, attitude towards work, job satisfaction, relationship with spouse, habit of having and spending money.

Case study will help student nurse to learn the techniques of making nursing assessment of the patient. Also will help her to make nursing diagnosis and plan for nursing intervention.

Important Test—A Nurse Should Know

1. Psychological test—are specialized assessment procedures for determining such a characteristic of an individual as intellectual capacity, motive pattern, self-concept, perception of environment, roles to be taken up, anxiety or depression, coping patterns and generally personality integration.
2. Intelligence tast—to assess intellectual abilities of patient. It has serious of task and problems. Such as matching geometrical designs, assembling the clock in a specific design.
3. Personality tests—help the clinical psychologist to evaluate patients feelings and personality structure.
4. Rorschach test, which consists of set of 10 inkblots. Patient is given one card at a time and asked to describe. What might this be? Or what does this remind you of?
5. Other test a patient is asked to create a story of what he perceives in the pictures. A patient is asked to draw a free-hand picture, psychologist interpret it. Questionnaire, which include three responses, true, false or cannot say. A large number of incomplete sentences given to patient and asked to complete them. The test helps in identifying the patients fears, goals or concerns, etc.

Psychiatric nurse faces various challenges because of changes in the patient care approach. She needs to update her knowledge in the field of psychiatric mental nursing. Staying in an urban community with lack of resources and ambitious goals, competitive spirit in the people is increasing, other types of stress such as housing, transport, lack of supplies, etc. the individual may not above to cope with the stress. Sudden change in the family system has brought changes in the life-style of the old people. Peer pressure especially on adolescent groups leads to various types of maladaptive behaviour like delinquency, dropouts, drug abuse, aids or behavior problems. They take up certain bad habits like alcoholism and excessive smoking, which leads to health problem.

Mass media, TV, computer and other electronic system have brought a lot of changes in the people. The impact of education is vivid and strong in the people when they watch or hear something.

Move forward with renewed determination and assess the challenges ahead of us. The only door one for us is to face the new challenges. What we require is action and courage. Nurses have established to credentials of nursing profession all over the world. Nursing profession has grown with times. Nurses are our countries lifeline. We have to shade away our outdated paths to explore and reach new world. Let us awake, arise and act. Nurses have been contributing immensely in the field. In this age of specialization, the multispecialty nature of nursing is coming to the force. Not to think that make you unfit.

Are the nurses educationally prepared to take up these challenges?

Are there any standards of psychiatric mental health nursing to maintain quality care? Ability to do research work and use findings for improvement of patient care.

Does Your Life Have A Purpose?

Are you contributing anything useful to this world of care? What is it lacking today? What would it take to get the missing ingredients into your life? How do you stick to your priorities?

Your thought affects your health. Health is never an issue until someone gets sick. Do not play with your health. The world you live in is created by your mind. A disease known is half cured. Health and wealth are state of mind. Be happy with who you are and what you have. Thoughts can make you more ill than any virtue.

Swami Vivekananda when he said the hands that help are holier than the lips that pray."

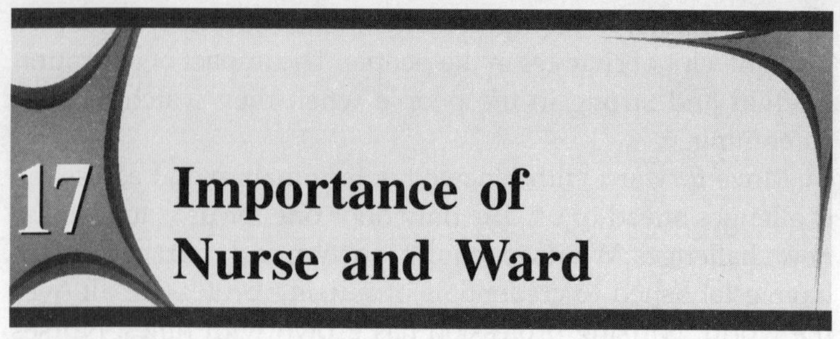

Importance of Nurse and Ward

MANAGERIAL SKILLS FOR NURSES

Hospital is an organization, where, nurses function at various hierarchical levels, set standard care to be provided, make plan on based resources available, assigns personnel to carry out plan, gives directions and controls their activities, evaluations according needs of patient and plan done weather implemented effectively. Evaluates work for improvement nursing care.

What is management?

Ward management:

Ward management is the responsibility of the head nurse and her nursing team. The ward management includes—
1. Management of patient care
2. Management of the personnel
3. Management of supplies and equipment
4. Management of environment
5. Careful plan the work—Hours of work, relieving persons
6. Organize the way it will be done
7. Who will do it decide
8. Control the quality of work done
9. Coordinate activities
10. Job description to apt personnel
11. Schedule the time hour of duty

12. Standardize routine procedures
13. Differentiate the heaviest days of work to light days
14. Determine special days of surgeries, doctor's rounds.

Good planning will build attitude, relationship and coordination among the staffs. If the patients are getting good nursing care, the people begin to understand what good nursing care means and how it is done.

MANAGEMENT OF PATIENT CARE ADMISSION AND ORIENTATION OF THE PATIENT

There are definite procedures prescribed by the hospital policies regarding the admission of the patient. Nurses should remember that for a patient and his relatives the hospital is a strange place and they need orientation by the nurses. Remember the proverb first impression is the best and lasting impression to the patient and his relatives. The new patient and his relatives should be oriented to—
1. The hospital as a whole (OPD, IPD) and to the particular ward or unit where he will be admitted to.
2. The routines of the hospital—Doctor's visiting time, visitor's visiting time, time for meals, etc.
3. Rules and regulations pertaining to the patient and his relatives.
4. Personnel working in the department and other patients admitted in the same department.
5. Ward equipment that may be used for the patient, e.g. a cardiac monitor.
6. Ward procedure.

Admission of the Patient

Admission of patient to the hospital can be traumatic experience with causing anxiety and fear for every person.
- Patient no longer enjoys the special privilege that of home.
- Most people are not used to hospital regimen and atmosphere.

- The person looses his identity and independence and control of daily activities.
- The nurse is the most important person the patient meet in the ward he admitted.
- She helps to diminish some of the fear and anxiety establishing trusting relationship as a nurse.
- The duration of severity of illness influences his reaction to the admission procedure.
- Also financial and economic problem too relation to his fear and anxiety.

Purpose of Admission

1. To receive him in the ward according to his condition
2. To provide comfort and safety
3. To welcome the patient
4. To provide immediate care
5. To be ready for any emergency
6. To assist his to adjust to new hospital environment
7. To obtain information about patient's contacts
8. Get information on any drug allergies, past diseases
9. To relieve fear and anxiety and encourage adjustment
10. Keep the bed room ready
11. Assemble necessary equipments
12. Introduce yourself
13. To know the condition of patient on admission
14. Assist the physician on level of treatment
15. Provide privacy and orientation.

ASSESSMENT OF THE PATIENT'S NEEDS AND PLANNING OF THE PATIENT'S CARE

As soon as the nurse comes in contact with patient, she should assess the needs of the patient and make a plan for his care. Maslow's hierarchy of needs can be a guide to provide for giving priority to these needs. The nurse makes use of every opportunity to collect necessary data for making diagnosis and nursing interventions. After collecting the data, she makes a plan for the care of the patient. The plan is made known to all the members of her team to provide continuity of the care. The important aspects of her planning should include—

1. To establish a patent airway and to ensure that the patient is breathing normally.
2. To check for adequate circulation and tissue perfusion (oxygenation).
3. To provide for the psychological support and meeting the spiritual needs.
4. To prevent the development of complication.
5. To support the activities of daily living such as mouth care, daily bath, bed shampoo, feeding, changing of cloths, elimination, etc.
6. To provide for continuous monitoring of the patient, such as checking of temperature, pulse, respiration, BP, I/O, mental status, elimination, skin color and integrity of the skin, etc.
7. To facilitate rehabilitation of the patient.
8. To educate the patient and his family in the area of their knowledge deficit.
9. To provide for the comfort of the patient by eliminating pain, insomnia, boredom, inactivity, etc.
10. To ensure safety for the patient.

Ward management is the responsibility of the head nurse and her nursing team. The ward management includes—

- Management of patient care
- Management of the personnel
- Management of supplies and equipment
- Management of environment.

Management is the art of getting the work done through and with the people in formally organized groups. It is cooperative effort directed towards laid down objectives.

Organized activities towards common objectives.

Good human relation that motivates people to function, leadership, communication, participation, dynamics core.

Process planning, organizing, coordinating controlling activities on order to archive objectives, reasons, activities, functions, outcome, thinking, doing.

Success Depends on Effectiveness and Efficacy of Management

Qualities

Good physique, health and vigorous moral, sense of discriminate right and wrong, a sense of responsibilities, general knowledge, technical knowledge of the work he supervising, experience of work.

Principles

Division of work assigns work to a person best suited.

Management—POSDCORB—Planning, organizing, staffing, directing, controlling, reporting and budgeting.

Authority and responsibility—authority without responsibility and responsibility without authority is useless.

Discipline—Obedience to authority, observe rules of service, respect.

Unity of command—Subordinate receives orders from one superior-would be confused-conflict in instructions.

Unity of directions—Two or more leaders—rivalries develop—competitions.

Subordination of individual interest and general interest, common interest.

Remuneration paid fair, satisfying.

Centralization of authority—A single person control authority. Authority divided in different persons control more effective.

Scalar chain—Hierarchy of authority line of workers purpose of communication proper channels chain.

Order-proper selection and placement of personnel.

Stability of tenure—Security of job.
Initiative—Think out plan and execute.
Union is strength, encourage among his employees.

Level of Management

Top chief executive, director, divisional head, sectional head superintendent.
Supervisory—Senior, front line, head nurse, senior staff nurse.

Management of Supplies and Equipment

1. Inadequate supply of materials—When there is inadequate number of pillows in ward; the patient cannot be position comfortably in bed.
2. The quality of nursing care is lowered down.
3. It endangers life of critically ill patient.
4. Treatment may be delayed.
5. The substitute e.g. instead of pillow sheet may be more costly, e.g. a rubber proof cover for a matters will prevent the matters from soiling an insufficient supply of syringes and needles may mean that they do not get properly sterilized results in infection.
   - Equipment may be out of order which causes an embarrassing situation to doctors and nurses when patient comes prepared for procedure.
   - Supplies and equipment may be inaccessibly—to prevent misuse, theft the articles are kept under lock and key. The key is misplaced, carried by chance, time wasted hunting.

If Articles are Kept in Several Scattered Room Wastage Of Time and Energy

1. Keep adequate supply at all times— in good working condition, in order, easily available, key available in ward all time and all know where it is kept, delegate responsibility to responsible person.
2. Regular and surprised checking of the inventory will help to maintain articles in good order.
3. Educate economic use of materials.
4. Use it in proper way in which it is designed to use.
5. Prevent wastage and misuse materials, maintenance, supplies and equipments.
6. Set a standard for quality of each item to be kept in the ward, e.g. Four pieces of 10, 2 ml syringes, if broken, lost replace but total number should not exceed.
7. The surgical need different items than orthopedic, children's ward' children need different items then elderly.
8. Men need different items than women.
9. ICU need emergency equipment.
10. Costly item to minimum.
11. Breakable stock large in quality same with perishable items.

System for Replacing/worn out Equipment

Replacement—Returned to store room before new articles is issued.

Specification, size, number, description. Count on monthly basis, weekly basis, and daily return borrowed articles.

Serial number- articles-specification-standard number- date of check up-sign of a person checked.

Management of environment—Ventilation, lighting, noise, unpleasant odor, dust control, safe disposal of excreta and waste, safe water supply, fire precaution, protection from radiation, privacy, cross infection control visitor, cleanliness, orderliness, insects.

Progressive Patient Care

This is organizing patient care units according to patient's needs for medical and nursing care instead of segregating patients, according to services—medical, surgical, gynecological, orthopedic, etc. patients are nursed in different units according to the degree of illness suffered by them. These progressive nursing care units are named as ICU, intermediate care units, self-care units, etc.

Intensive care units— The critically ill patients, such as those suffering from coronary thrombosis, cardiorespiratory failure, and cerebral vascular accidents, patients who are undergoing major surgery and other patients who need constant attention are admitted to the ICU.

The purpose of ICU is life saving. All kinds of emergency equipments necessary for the resuscitation of the patients are available in these units. Each unit has the provision for administering oxygen, suction, continuous monitoring of BP, pulse, respirations, body temperature, cardiac functioning, etc. sufficient skilful help is available both day and night.

Here the patient is under the constant observation by the nurses who are highly skilled and experience in the care of critically ill patients. The medical attention by the doctors also will be available all through 24 hours.

Intermediate Care Units

When the patient no longer need the close attention by the nurses they are transferred to the intermediate care units. Here the patients have the continuity of care which they were receiving in the ICU.

Self-Care Units

Most of the patients in the self-care units are ambulatory. The patients who are recovered from critically ill diseases and are ready to of to home or those who are admitted for investigations are seen in there units. The workload in these units is very less compared to other units.

Priority Nursing Care

The saving of a life depends on promptness of action. Do the first tings first is the golden rule for a successful nursing care. We find that the patient may be suffering from different health problems some of them are endangering the life of the patient.

In order to save the patient, these problems should be dealt with quickly, e.g. failure of breathing, severe bleeding, severe shock, etc., every moment is precious. When a patient is brought to the hospital, the nurse observes that his breathing is failing, he has injury on the head and the wound is bleeding and the patient is severely dehydrated. The nurse gives priority to the breathing problems, then to the bleeding and then to the dehydration present in the patient.

Abraham Maslow's hierarchy of need is helpful in determining priorities. He described pyramid of needs with primary or physiologic needs at the base and the secondary or nonphysiologic needs at the higher levels. It is assumed that the physiological needs should always be given a higher priority then other needs on the hierarchy—the life-threatening crises take precedence over everything else. However, when setting priorities, individual circumstances and desires of each patient must be considered.

Assignment of Personnel for Patient Care

When the nurse has made the plan of care, she needs right personnel for the implementation of her plan. When she has selected the right personnel she delegates the responsibilities with authority. The assignment of the personnel will be done in three ways—

The Functional Method: The work is divided among the personnel and each person is concerned with a particular task. For example one nurse may take tap, gives all the injections and medications and does all the charting. Other nurses may serve the diets and maintains the intake output of all the patients. Another may give bath and related morning care. Another may prepare the patient for special procedures and treatments. Another person may make beds, records, admissions and discharges, keeps charts in order, etc.

The functional method of assignment has several disadvantages and advantages. It is believed to be more economical of time and effort. It is a simple way of getting the assigned according to the qualification and experience of the personnel. The tasks which require less attention may be entrusted with junior nurses or nurses with less experience.

There is danger in using the functional method of assignment that individual needs of the patient are lost in an effort to gte the ward work done. One cannot say, who will be really responsible for the patient and the patient will not have the confidence to open his problems to anyone. No one nurse will know completely about the patient. It is likely that each nurse may assume that another has done particular functions which are not entrusted to her. With there result, the patient feels that he is neglected. The nurses became task oriented and not person oriented, hence the patient becomes neglected.

The Patient Method of Assignment

In this method, the head nurses assign the total care of a group of patients to each personnel in the ward. Each personnel are responsible for complete care of each patient assigned to her, regardless of her abilities and experience.

If this method is to function efficiently, the head nurse has to arrange the patient in carefully selected groups, so that each group consists of different categories of patients. Such as completely bed ridden, partially bedridden, convalescent and ambulant patients. If this arrangement is not made one nurse may have all the bedridden patients, another will have all ambulant patients and this makes lot of work difference in the workload.

Actually ill patient, demanding, patients using extra equipments, patient with some extra nursing care problems, e.g. incontinence of urine or stool, paralysis patient, etc. patient who need constant supervision, patient who is under shock, need more time than other patient who are ambulant, chronically ill, etc.

In order to distribute the workload equally among the personnel, these patients should be placed in such a way that there will be mixing of seriously ill patients with ambulant. Patient is also an important factor. If these patients are placed in close proximity to one another and to the service units, much less time is spent by the nurses in going from one to another.

This method has several disadvantages also. The personnel with high personnel abilities and experience and the personnel with less personnel abilities and experience require doing the same type of tasks. When there is shortage of staffs, the care of patients are divided among the available staff regardless of patients needs or personnel abilities. The greatest advantage of this method of assignment is that it helps to establish a nurse-patient relationship.

The nursing team method of assignment—has advantages over both the functional and the patient methods of assignment. The team method of assignment developed from a need to utilize the knowledge and skills of the staff nurse to better advantage, and to ensure the supervision of axillary nursing personnel.

The concept of nursing team is based on the philosophy has a group of nursing personnel working together in a coordinated, cooperative way, can carry out the full functions of nurse in giving the patient individual care.

The nursing team is usually composed of both qualified and nonqualified personnel. All the nursing team will have a team leader, who is an experience staff nurse and one or more member of the auxiliary nursing staff. The head nurse makes the assignments of patients and the personnel to the team leader.

The teamleader plans the nursing care and each patient and assigns the care of patients to the member's of her team. She reserves for herself the full responsibilities for the care of critically ill patients or patients who presents special problems. The nursing team method of assignment has several advantages.

It allow the team leader to use her knowledge, ability and skills in analyzing, planning and giving individualized nursing care of patient.

It releases her from tasks which misuses her time and energy.

It places her in a position which allows her to know and understand the needs of her patient.

It allows the head nurse to contribute her expert guidance for the whole patients under her custody.

The nurse develop good interpersonal relationship among them by working cooperatively, develop supervisory and leadership qualities.

The non professional team members have greater sense of importance and of belongings because their contributions are recognized. They are given more responsibility and they receive more supervision and instruction.

The head nurse has time to study many problems arising in the management of patient care and the personnel management and is able to tackle there problems efficiently.

The team method of patient assignment results in improvement of patient care through personalized and compassionate consideration of his needs as a patient and as a person and through full utilization of all members of the nursing staff.

The team leader improves her managerial skills. In order to assign the patients, first of all she has to analyze the needs of each patient and then she must make an assessment of the abilities of each member of her team, in order to ensure that the patients are placed in expert hands for the nursing care.

Its disadvantages imply that the same group is working together consistently. Team cannot function unless there is a stable staff. Unless the team leader develops leadership qualities, she will not be able to plan, organize and supervise the work of the personnel working in her team.

Nurse-patient ratio-ICU 1: 1 per shift
3 nurses 24 hours for a patient.

In intermediate care units, the staffing strength varies with shift. In the morning shift it may be one. Nurse for 3-5 patients in the evening shift it one to 7 patients, and in the night one: 11patients.

Planning a time schedules and work schedules is useful administrative devices for the orderly regulation of activities and for avoiding omissions.

Objectives—
To provide adequate nursing care 24 hours each.
To promote good relationship and satisfaction among personnel.
The work schedule outlines the basic duties of the various grades of personnel. These are usually written in order of sequence of work as far as possible. The technique of job analysis is of great help in the competition of time and work schedule.
For example of a work schedule for the head nurse daily program.

Ward-
Name-
Time schedule-

7 to 7.30 planning assignments for the staff, students and other
Getting reports from night nurse.
Providing enough supplies and equipment.
Sending for repairs and refilling.

7-8 am orientation of new staff

8-8.30 making round in the patients ward.
Getting ready for doctors round.

10.30-10.45 coffee break.

10.45-12 noon supervising the activities of the nursing students
Conducting ward teaching programme.

12-12. 30 conference with the staff.

12.30-1 pm short round in the ward.
Checking the effects of treatment.

1-1.30 lunch break.

1.30-2.30 completing the reports and records.
Evaluation of the days work.
Preparing for the handing over to the personnel of next shift.
Checking inventory.
Helping patient for afternoon rest.

2.30-2.45 making a short round in the ward.
Expediting any work that undone.

2.45-3 pm handing over duties to the personnel of the next shift.

Sample of the Weekly Program for the Head Nurse

1. Planning the working hours, duty assignment for the staff, students and others.
2. Sending breakages, losses and getting them replaced.
3. Indenting new supplies in the ward.
4. See to the general cleanliness of ward.
5. Arranging ward teaching programme for the staff and students.
6. Arranging for the ward conferences.
7. Evaluation of the weeks program.
8. Supervision of the performance of the evening and night staff.

Sample of the Monthly Program for the Head Nurse

1. Planning of ward teaching for the student.
2. Planning of in-service programme for the staff.
3. Checking the inventory, drugs, etc.
4. Arranging conference for the staff, nursing students and others.
5. Writing and sending evaluation of the staff and students.

Samples of the Yearly Program for the Head Nurse

1. Planning for general cleanliness of the ward (white washing, painting).
2. Sending annual demands for furniture, equipments, etc.
3. Arranging for the medical check up of the staff and nursing students, etc.
4. Helping in the annual examination of the student.

Weekly Time Schedule

Name- job title-Monday to Sunday-day-evening-night

Time schedules need to be written at least for a week. The name of the each staff member should be listed with their designation, e.g. head nurse, staff nurse, hospital aid, etc.

The hours of duty and the days of leave are indicated against the names, every day, from Monday to Sunday.

The nurses who relieve the other nurses should be clearly known.

It is helpful when the number of staff for each shift is shown at the bottom of the schedule.

The total of each shift at the bottom of the schedule immediately shows the shortage of staff in any shift on any day.

A master plan for a month may be prepared which will help to space and rotate the days off.

When a number of staff change duty on the same day, it is good, if all the available staff can be on duty.

When there is a change of shift, it is better to change the duty to the previous shift that is the night staff.

Change their duty with the evening staff, the staff in the evening shift changes their duty with the morning shift and the staff in the morning shift; change their duty with the night shift.

This will give adequate time interval between their shifts and there will be enough personnel in the ward for duty.

The attitudes, relationships and cooperation among the staff will be much better, if they are given some choice in their day off.

Principles of Time Planning and Patient Assignments

1. Consider the busy days and less busy days.
2. Equal distribution of task for all personnel is important.
3. Consider the qualification and experience of personnel while assigning duties.
4. Plan the time off and duty hours in such a way as to have enough personnel in the ward.
5. Overlap the duty hours for continuity of the work.
6. Trainees should be working with the trained personnel.
7. Plan the day off for the nursing students when there is no class.
8. Consider the special requests made by the personnel, whenever possible.
9. When there is not adequate numbers of personnel, mix the seriously ill patients with moderately ill patients.

WARD ROUND

- The head nurse makes two types of ward rounds.
- The ward rounds made with physician and the ward rounds made by her or with the nursing staff.
- The ward rounds made with the physician are to diagnoses disease and to prescribe the treatment in the care of patients.
- Since the head nurse is responsible for the ward management, she has several purposes for a ward rounds, they are—

1. To observe the physical and mental condition of the patient and the progress made day by day.
2. To observe the work of the staff.
3. To make specific observation of the patient and to give report to the doctor, e.g. Wounds, dressing, drainage, bleeding, etc.
4. To introduce the patients to the personnel and the personnel to the patients.
5. To carry out the plan made for the care of the patients.
6. To observe the results of treatment and the satisfaction of the patient with his care.
7. To ensure the safety measures employed for the safety of the patient and the personnel.
8. To give recreational and divisional therapy for he patient
9. To meet the spiritual needs of the patient.
10. To teach the nursing students and the hospital aids' to check any preventable conditioned present in the patient such as bed sores, foot drops, etc.
11. To check the emergency equipments kept near patient and to check their safety and working order.
12. To observe the cleanliness of the ward, sanitary annexes, etc.
13. To take over and hand over the duties at the change of shifts.
14. To expedite the work left undone:
    - When doctor's round is expected the head nurse collect all the available information relevant to each patient.
    - She sees that all charts are up to date.
    - The latest reports and X-rays are kept ready for inspection she will be able to give an accurate report of all patients in the ward, e.g. if she has to report about diabetic patient she has to study the results and 4 hourly urine testing, the amount of insulin patient is taking daily, any signs of hypoglycemia after insulin.
    - The type of diet, total calorie, fluid, weight, infections.
    - As a preparation for rounds, she prepares and keeps ready all those equipment that are likely to be asked such as BP instrument, diagnostic set, flash light, etc.

- A doctor always finds it very annoying to have to at wait the nurse prepares the tray or goes to another department to bring an equipment.
- The nurse, who is responsible to go for round, keeps equipment ready or to position the patient for the physical examination.
- She sends visitors away prior to round to prevent any disturbances that may occurs during the round.
- Correct position of head nurse accompanying doctor is patients, left side-doctor on right side.
- Which helps any help necessary for examination of the patient, e.g. to undress patient to position it helps her to give attention to the doctor when he gives order.
- Immediately after the round, the head nurse should be prompt to carry out the doctor's order.
- Any delay makes the patient to become impatient.

Reports and Record

A report is one form and orientation because it is purpose is to impart information about the exiting situation, therefore it is used to prepare the personnel for their days work. Complete and consist reports are vital for good —management and administration. No team can function efficiently without this method of communication. Every nurse should have thoroughly knowledge of the patient's condition, including his problems, treatment and day-to-day progress which will give at glance information. Orally/written. It is an art. Give proper time when patient came turn over other to another.

This constant exchange of information is essential to provide good patient care.

24 Hours Report

It gives informations of all patients in ward that is total number of patients, their names, diagnosis, seriously ill, new admissions, operated, scheduled for surgery, those discharge or transferred from the ward.

Samples of an Accident Report

Name, age, ward number, bed number, address, OPD number, place, date and time of accident.
Description of how the accident occurred.
Safety, precaution, condition of the patient before and after the accident.
Doctor's examination findings.
Treatment ordered.
Witness to accident—name and address.
Signature of doctor.
Signature of the nurse.
Unit.
Date and report.

Management of Emergencies

- At any time, medical emergencies may arise that require immediate resuscitation of the patient.
- The nursing team should be prepared to meet any type of emergency.
- They should keep the unit ready at all times with equipment, supplies and drugs for immediate resuscitation of the patient, so that no time is lost to initiate the treatment.
- The nurses may follow the standing orders and the policies of the hospital to resuscitate the patient while waiting for the doctor's arrival.
- They should know how to get the medical aid, who to call for help and what to do immediately to resuscitate the patient.

Patient Teaching

Every patient has the right to know the nature of his illness, its prognosis, its treatment, its preventative, promotive and rehabilitative aspects, the health problems that he may have to face in the future. The relatives also should be aware of these facts in order to help the patient.

The patient teaching should be started with the admission the patient and it should be continued throughout his stay in the hospital and even after his discharge from the hospital.

It should be regular features of his rehabilitation program.

As a part of the teaching program, certain procedures may be taught to the patient before his discharge from the hospital.

For example diabetic patient may be taught the technique of taking insulin injection.

Patient teaching can be formal or incidental and may be given individual or group. Can distribute printed literature on various aspects of health care.

Following Principles While Health Education

1. Introduce only one subject at a time.
2. Contents should have logical sequences that is start from the simple to difficult, from known to unknown facts.
3. Use only technique terms.
4. Ask the patient to repeat the information to ensure understanding of patient.
5. Use AV aids whenever possible.

Appraisal of Nursing Services

Periodic evaluation of the nursing services of nursing care, the focus—

1. Structure—Physical facilities, equipment and supplies, staffing, etc.
2. Process-nursing techniques, nursing procedures, quantity and quality of care, adequacy and appropriateness of care.
3. Outcome—Patients satisfaction, satisfaction of personnel engaged in the patient care, lower accident and complication rates promptness in the performance of the term meeting the objectives and the policies of the hospital.

Management of the Personnel

- Orientation of the new personnel.
- The initial orientation of the new personnel should be done by the nursing administration.
- The new person taken in a tour of the entire hospital to see its facilities.
- She is introduced to every department and its personnel.
- Explain about organization of the hospital, the line of authority, the channels of communication, the hospital policies, etc.

Supervision of Personnel and Delegations of Responsibility

Type of supervision depends upon the leadership styles of the head nurse. Autocratic and free rein form of supervision is desirable because it pays attention to the person as well as the work.

Points-Head Nurse

1. Make sure that the subordinate knows how to do the work assigned to her. She should be told what, when, where, why, who and how of the job. Good orientation will help in this area.
2. Assign the responsibility with no overlapping when two people are assigned to do the same job, there is danger that each will rely on the other to perform the entire task, with the result that neither does. It should be clear what is assigned to each one.
3. Delegate responsibility with authority. Authority should equal to responsibility.
4. Specify clearly the duties, responsibilities and relationship of each job. Job description will help in this matter.
5. Consider each work of a individual. It is not sufficient to divide the total amount of work among the total number of personnel. To make a good assignment, consider each

work as an individual and make the assignment based on such factors as—
- Her professional qualification
- Her previous experience
- Her personal qualities
- Her technical; competence.

6. Consider that total workload assigned— It is not possible for a nurse to take BP every 15 minutes on one patient and to care for another. Who is in isolation. Neither can she care for two patients who require constant observation re-located in different rooms.
7. Consider the supervision available for each personnel. A new personnel require more supervision than a person who is in the unit for a longer period.
8. Plans should be flexible enough to include unforeseen events. A surgical patient may start to bleed; a patient may go in cardiac arrest who needs resuscitation immediately. Therefore all the plans may not be implemented according to the original schedule.
9. Periodical evaluation of the performance of each member is essential. No assignment is complete until one is satisfied that it has achieved its objectives.

Establishment of Interpersonal Relationship (IPR)

The head nurse is in key position for the establishment of good IPR among the personnel in her department. This will also involve communication system existing between and within the hospital departments. A warm, friendly attitude of nurses is reflected to patient and other employee.

Point IPR

1. Every member should be kept informed about the job, any changes that are taking place from day-to-day/ effective communication.
2. Give personnel recognition to everyone by giving praise and showing concern whenever they deserve.

3. Know each personnel working with you and accept them with there abilities and limitations.
4. Any grievances should be dealt with promptly and appropriately.
5. Do not do or say anything that will lower the status of the member in your team.
6. Plan, organize and coordinate the activities of your team, so that everything gets done in the proper time and in the correct way.
7. Remember that every member of your team is working with you and not for you or under you.
8. Try to create we feeling in your subordinate.
9. Give each person time and opportunity to plan his work and make sure that everyone understand the work assigned to her.
10. Provide adequate supplies and equipment needed in the patient care.
11. Except in time of emergency avoid interrupting personnel while they are at work.
12. Plan for frequent staff conference.

Evaluation of Personnel

Valuation should be done as many times as necessary. It helps in giving promotion, incentives, and transfer. It helps to improve the quality of service.

The Qualities Assessed

1. Qualities of performance/skills.
2. Mental qualities.
3. Personal, supervisory qualities.
4. Capacity for further development. To give worthwhile results.

Staff Conference and Purpose

1. It is vital for the success of patient care. Any problem that comes across in the care of patient in the maintenance of supplies and equipments, etc.
2. It helps to build up the group morale and IPR in the personnel.
3. I acts as a means of communication among the members of the working team.
4. It helps to up date the knowledge of the team members.
5. It helps in decision-making and problem solving.

Select a time and a place that does not conflict with the work of other personnel. Staff conferences are held as frequently as possible. It need not be lengthy. Always start the conference in time. Keeps the discussion moving forward towards a solution? Encourage all the members of a team to participate in the discussion. Utilize all the opportunities for making clarifications demonstrations, teachings, etc. always prepare an agenda that is to be discussed in the conference.

Staff development program—CME (Continuous Medical Education) which helps the individual to maintain and improve her skills in the current job and prepares her for possible promotion.

Training courses, seminars and workshops outside the institution.

Health safety and welfare—preemployment examination physical exam, periodic re-examination, health education to develop health habits, hygiene, hazards, infection, provide recreation facilities, employ counseling benevolent funds retirement plans, provision of rest room, canteen and living facilities.

Planning— is one of the major fundamental element of administration. It is a process of setting guidelines. It sketches a complete mental picture, it is comprehensive integrative process determines future course of action to achieve desired results. It should be simple, focus on purpose, precise, provide resources and always documented. It is characterized by continuity, and flexibility.

All professional nurse staffs- in critical cases unit, PT, labor unit and emergency room keep nurse patient ratio, empower head nurse reward employees. Use of scientific tests for determining abilities of the candidates. Taping capable candidate and placing in right job. There is always a shortage of nursing for high quality care.

Salary, insurance benefits, CME opportunities made available for a better future. Her ability, intelligence, aptitude and personality rewarded. Experience, seniority, initiative, particular knowledge is considered in promotion.

Life saving is the priority, assisting human needs for faster recovery and rehabilitation. The workload connected with human beings is never constant. Human needs are varied at varied stressful situation. Who are with patient round the clock? Nursing plays vital roles in safeguarding the health of the people.

Nursing needs to develop in its potentialities as millions are in need of expert care by nurses. Nurses lose their cool in a constant stress ridden environment due to over crowding with patient and relatives and deplorable working conditions. After all there is some limit to human endurance.

Nature of Nursing Administration

A technical knowledge of a field which enables the administrator to perform her tasks. coordinating efforts of people; so that they can work together to accomplish their set tasks. Accomplish common goals, e.g. public health and building of bridges. The process is dynamic and creative universal and holistic on going process, social and human, creative and innovative consists of structure.

Management is an agency which directs and guides. Organization aims towards specific objective and goals. It can be applicable to all walks of life. It has to be therefore smooth functioning of schools, colleges, hospitals, health centers and public and private enterprises. It includes formulation of objectives, plan and policies. Management is executive function responsible for translating those formulated plans, policies and procedures into action to achieve goals.

Division of work—Cannot perform all activities to achieve its objectives. Accountability and responsibility, discipline, unity of command, unity of direction, fair policy, collective bargaining, initiative, and stability are some of the principles.

Word 'POSDCORD'— Planning, Organizing, Staffing, Directing, Coordinating, Reporting, Budgeting are elements of administration.

Observing workers performance selecting best worker, training selected worker, paying, motivating highly skilled worker to managerial position.

All activities in an organization should be technical, commercial, financial, security, accounting and administrative.

Index